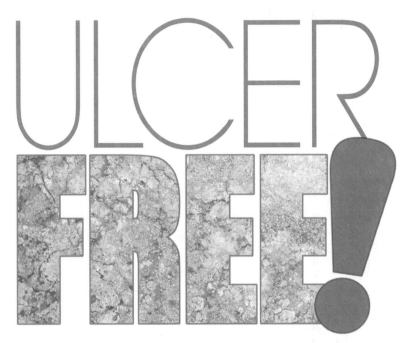

ULCER FREE!

Nature's Safe & Effective
REMEDY for ULCERS

GEORGES M. HALPERN, MD, PhD

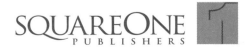

SQUAREONE
PUBLISHERS

The information and advice in this book are based on the training, personal experiences, and research of the author. Its contents are current and accurate; however, the information presented is not intended to substitute for professional medical advice. The author and the publisher urge you to consult with your physician or other qualified health-care provider prior to starting any treatment or undergoing any surgical procedure. Because there is always some risk involved, the author and publisher cannot be responsible for any adverse effects or consequences resulting from the use of any of the suggestions, preparations, or procedures described in this book.

COVER DESIGNER: Phaedra Mastrocola
IN-HOUSE EDITOR: Elaine Kennedy
TYPESETTER: Gary A. Rosenberg

Square One Publishers
115 Herricks Road
Garden City Park, NY 11040
(516) 535-2010 • (877) 900-BOOK
www.squareonepublishers.com

Library of Congress Cataloging-in-Publication Data
Halpern, Georges M.
    Ulcer free! : nature's safe & effective remedy for ulcers /
Georges M. Halpern.
       p. ; cm.
    Includes bibliographical references and index.
    ISBN 0-7570-0253-6
    1. Peptic ulcer—Popular works. 2. Carnosine—Therapeutic use—
Popular works.
    [DNLM: 1. Peptic Ulcer—etiology. 2. Peptic Ulcer—therapy. 3. Anti-Ulcer
Agents—therapeutic use. 4. Complementary Therapies. 5. Organometallic
Compounds—therapeutic use. WI 350 H195u 2004] I. Title.
RC821.H34   2004
616.3'4306—dc22

                                                                                    2004002479

Printed in the United States of America

10   9   8   7   6   5   4   3   2   1

Contents

*I dedicate this book to all patients who suffer
from the all-too-real pains of gastric disorders.
I hope this book will help them learn more
about their problem, and seek lasting relief.*

Acknowledgments

I would like to take this opportunity to thank those who helped turn the idea of this book into a reality: Anthony Almada, who connected me to Dan Murray; Dan, who provided a wealth of information and friendly support; and, Rudy Shur and Elaine Kennedy at Square One Publishers, who polished the words and published this book. I would also like to acknowledge and thank Peter Weverka—without whose talent and skill this project would not have been possible.

And last, but certainly not least, my wife Emiko who put up with me during the very stressful "book incubation" period.

Introduction

My interest in peptic ulcer disease is personal. I had a peptic ulcer. The year was 1962. I was chief resident in the maternity ward of a big city hospital just outside the center of Paris. Shifts lasted 36 hours. Between consultations, we performed a few Cesarean sections. On many occasions we saved the lives of poor, desperate women who had suffered at the hands of back-alley abortionists—at that time, abortion procedures were illegal. We also delivered babies whose mothers had been referred to us by midwives because they considered the births too risky.

Getting any sleep was out of the question, and even when I managed to string together a few precious hours of shut-eye, they were usually interrupted by Gerard Zwang, a fellow doctor and the future author of *Feminine Sexuality*, who was even then researching his sexology masterpiece with the aid of vocal female partners on the other side of the paper-thin wall next to which I slept, or at least tried to sleep. The doctor who was the head of the maternity ward was a closet morphine addict. He actually forbade my colleagues and me from giving anesthetic or tetanus shots to our patients. It was a most stressful time.

The food I managed to eat on the run was nondescript. The red wine I drank made coppers shine and my stomach cringe. I smoked a pack a day of non-filtered cigarettes. The chief resident in cardiology managed to melt the engine of my prized crimson Simca-1000. He forgot to check the oil and never noticed the fumes gushing out of the back of the car. I learned later that the man had

1

no sense of smell. And to top things off, I was going through a very painful divorce.

My ulcer pain was rhythmic. Like clockwork, it occurred four hours after each so-called meal I ate on the run. I controlled the pain with bismuth, my stomach medication of choice. An upper GI X-ray series confirmed my suspicions: it was an ulcer. "Second duodenum; quite unusual," mumbled the radiologist. I kept on swallowing my bismuth subnitrate not knowing that it had the potential to induce severe brain damage. I injected myself with a concoction of vitamin C and iron that was horribly painful.

In October of that year, I was drafted into the army. At the Château de Vincennes, an impressive dark castle on the outskirts of Paris that occasionally served as a state prison, I asked the physician on duty for some painkilling bismuth. This doctor was counting the minutes until his return to civilian life, but he managed to give me enough attention to notice my ulcer pain. After some initial tests, he called an ambulance. I was transported to a military hospital, where I got a gastroscopy with a rigid tube, quite different from the flexible tubes of today, another series of X-rays, more bismuth, and a confirmation of my diagnosis. I was relieved of my military duties. The training ship on which I was supposed to have been the physician on board left port without me on a twenty-month cruise around the world.

Forty-two years later, the scar from my peptic ulcer is still visible on barium X-ray pictures. I stopped smoking thirty years ago. I eat—as much as possible—great food at regular hours and drink only superb wines. I am happily married. I love my life between the house in Northern California and my job in Asia. But I know what ulcer pain feels like. I shall always know. That is why I have written this book. After decades of making sure I was familiar with the latest medical discoveries in ulcer treatments, I have found a simple, nontoxic, natural approach to relieving ulcer pain and treating ulcers.

While I may not have been the one to actually make the discovery, I am pleased to provide the first guide to this remarkable nutrient. For nearly a decade, Zinc-Carnosine has been effectively used in Japan to treat peptic ulcer disease and other gastrointestinal complaints. The supplement has been nothing short of miraculous in its ability to bolster the stomach's natural defenses and relieve ulcer pain and suffering. As both a teacher and physician, it would be imprudent to claim that this nutrient cures ulcers for every patient who takes it, but this unique supplement undoubtedly plays a significant healing role for most. For that reason, I believe that ulcer patients should know about Zinc-Carnosine. In this book, I present studies and the latest medical thinking about the supplement. I show why Zinc-Carnosine deserves a place beside prescription drugs as a treatment option for ulcer pain and ulcer disease. I show how Zinc-Carnosine may help prevent gastric ulcers.

As you will discover, this book is more than just a simple guide to Zinc-Carnosine. It has been designed to provide the reader with a look at both the problems of gastric diseases and the treatments currently used. Chapter 1 explains what an ulcer is and gives a history of ulcer treatments. Chapters 2, 3, and 4 examine the causes of peptic ulcer disease. Chapter 2 looks at the most common cause of ulcers—the bacterium *Helicobacter pylori* (*H. pylori*). It explains how *H. pylori* infects the stomach lining, and how and why certain people get ulcers from it. Chapter 3 describes how non-steroidal anti-inflammatory drugs (NSAIDs) erode the stomach lining, why these drugs are so useful in spite of the damage they do to the stomach, and how scientists are trying to modify NSAIDs so that patients can take them without risk. Chapter 4 looks at the causes of ulcer disease—stress, smoking, alcohol, and others—that usually fall under the ambiguous "lifestyle" heading.

Chapter 5 investigates ulcer symptoms and explains all the different diagnostic techniques, their costs and side effects, and why doctors choose one technique over the other.

The next three chapters take up ulcer treatments. Chapter 6 looks at standard drug treatments and antibiotic treatments for *H. pylori* infections, the drugs' side effects, how accurate different treatments are, and why doctors choose different treatments for their patients. Chapter 7 examines a handful of natural supplements and folk remedies for peptic ulcer disease. Chapter 8 brings readers up to date on Zinc-Carnosine, the novel ulcer treatment that I believe should be an option for everyone who is being treated for peptic ulcer disease and for those who believe that they are candidates for getting an ulcer.

Throughout this book, I have tried my best to explain medical procedures and gastrointestinal physiology in plain terms that everyone can understand. Besides being an adept listener, I believe a good doctor is one who can explain treatments and treatment options to patients in such a way that patients can understand what they are being told. I have endeavored to be a good doctor on the pages of this book.

If you stumble across a term you don't understand, I invite you to look it up in the glossary at the end of this book. Also at the end of this book, listed chapter by chapter, are references to the various studies that I have investigated.

In spite of improved diagnostic techniques and treatments, I know that far too many Americans suffer from peptic ulcer disease. Too many people are awakened in the middle of the night by crippling ulcer pain or the pain of another gastrointestinal disorder. Too many people have to abstain from the foods they like and the activities they enjoy in the interest of nursing their ulcer. It is my hope that once you have read this book, you will be able to talk intelligently with your doctor and decide on a treatment plan that is right for you. It is also my hope that this book will allow patients to take the right steps in their lives to avoid forever the tremendous pain and discomfort ulcer sufferers know too well.

1

Peptic Ulcer Disease

I t's early morning. The burning pain in your gut wakes you up before the alarm clock does. You knew you shouldn't have eaten that spicy food for dinner, but you couldn't resist. You go to the bathroom, down a few antacids, and you're ready to conquer the universe. You grab a donut and some coffee on your way to work, and your day begins. At about 10AM, the pain returns. You make it to lunch, but before you sit down in the cafeteria, you go to the pharmacy and replenish your supply of antacids. The pain subsides.

It's now around 3 PM. You're at a meeting, and again, you feel that burning sensation in the pit of your stomach. You make a mental note to definitely skip the fries at lunch tomorrow as you grab another antacid from your pocket. How prepared are you? By the end of the day, you've consumed half-a-dozen antacids and made a promise to yourself at bedtime to change your eating habits . . . really! What you don't know is that your body is telling you something—and no matter what you've done to stop it from communicating with you, the damage is progressing.

For millions of people living in North America, this story is all too common. What they don't know is that their peptic ulcers are masquerading as heartburn, bloating, acid reflux, and other gastric problems. While they self-medicate with a host of over-the-counter (OTC) products to relieve the pain, the underlying problem remains, and in most instances, worsens as time goes by. How widespread is the problem? It is estimated that 4.5 million people suffer from peptic ulcers. This also explains why antacids constitute the number-one category of best-selling OTC preparations in drugstores.

If you think you have a peptic ulcer or your doctor has confirmed this condition, this book is for you. It will provide you with important information that will make you a more active participant in your course of treatment, and it will provide you with options you may not know exist. In this chapter, I will lay the groundwork for the rest of the book. I examine the prevalence of peptic ulcer disease in the United States—in other words, you are not alone. I explain what ulcers are, their symptoms, and their complications. I explain why ulcers sometimes fail to heal. Finally, this chapter offers a brief and selective look at the history of ulcer treatments.

IMPACT OF PEPTIC ULCER DISEASE

According to the American Gastroenterological Association, 25 million Americans will get an ulcer in their lifetime. Annually, 4.5 million Americans suffer from ulcer disease. Peptic ulcers affect 11 to 14 percent of American men and 8 to 11 percent of American women. Depending on the study you read, there are approximately 350,000 to 500,000 new cases annually. About 6,000 people die each year from ulcer-related complications. Contrary to popular belief, your occupation or social class does not increase or decrease your chances of getting an ulcer.

In real terms, the statistics just given indicate that an extraordinary number of Americans are suffering with peptic ulcer disease. Some patients are bedridden for a week at a time. They have to miss days of work and often are unable to engage in physical activity or exercise. In one survey, 40 percent of ulcer patients reported having to see a physician five or more times in the course of a year. Visiting the doctor, not to mention purchasing medications, can be costly. Patients have to be careful what they eat and avoid foods that irritate their stomachs. Their sleep is interrupted by ulcer pain. Because ulcer pain comes and goes, they never know from moment to moment when ulcer pain will accost or cripple them.

The following statistics give an overall picture of the public and private costs of treating peptic ulcer disease in the United States:

- More than 1 million Americans are hospitalized each year for an ulcer-related illness.

- The cost of lost time at work and lack of productivity is about $500 million annually.

- The collective cost to individuals for treating peptic ulcers is $5 billion to $10 billion annually.

- Treating peptic ulcers costs taxpayers approximately $2 billion per year.

The statistics are grim, but, mercifully, physician visits and hospitalization rates for peptic ulcer disease have been steadily declining since the 1960s, thanks to improved diagnostic methods and better treatments. Today, the mortality rate is slightly over one death per 100,000 people—one-third of what the rate was twenty-five years ago. In the years since 1970, advances in the treatment of peptic ulcer disease have eclipsed and rendered obsolete most of the treatments and diagnostic techniques of the past. If it's any consolation, now is the best time in human history to have a peptic ulcer. What concerns doctors, however, are the hospitalization rates for hemorrhaging and perforated ulcers. These rates have remained the same or, in the case of stomach ulcers, have risen dramatically due to the increased use of non-steroidal anti-inflammatory drugs (NSAIDs) in the elderly population.

The use of NSAIDs by the elderly is changing the face of peptic ulcer disease in the United States and other industrialized countries. *H. pylori* infection remains the primary cause of peptic ulcer disease throughout the world, but in industrialized countries where good sanitary conditions prevail and bacteria are not as catching, the use of NSAIDs will probably surpass *H. pylori* infections as the primary cause within a generation or two. In industrialized countries, with people living longer, more are afflicted by such diseases of old age as arthritis and osteoporosis, which require taking NSAIDs to relieve pain. Australia offers an excellent example of the connection between NSAIDs and ulcer disease in

NSAIDs

You are going to hear a lot about NSAIDs, or non-steroidal anti-inflammatory drugs, in this book. Whether you know it or not, you are probably not a stranger to NSAIDs. Ninety-five percent of Americans have at least one type of NSAID in their medicine cabinet. The most popular NSAID is aspirin. Ibuprofen (brand names Advil, Motrin) is also an NSAID. People take these drugs to relieve pain and decrease tissue swelling, but if they are taken persistently over a long period of time, they can cause peptic ulcers. I explain how NSAIDs cause ulcers, the drugs' many side effects, and other issues concerning NSAIDs in Chapter 3.

developed countries. In the nine years between 1979 and 1988, Australia saw a twofold increase in the consumption of non-aspirin NSAIDs, and, not coincidentally, a twofold increase in the number of people over 65 with stomach ulcers.

As people live longer, they will take more NSAIDs and acquire peptic ulcers more frequently. And many elderly people will have to continue taking their NSAIDs in spite of their ulcers. These drugs are absolutely essential to people who suffer from crippling arthritic pain. By taking Zinc-Carnosine, elderly ulcer sufferers can guard the lining of the stomach from the corrosive effects of non-steroidal anti-inflammatory drugs.

WHAT IS A PEPTIC ULCER?

Before we look at peptic ulcers, let's explain what an ulcer is. Any small portion of the skin or surface of an internal tissue can develop inflammation. This affected area of inflammation is called a lesion. In its early stage, it can have the appearance of a second-degree burn with reddening, blistering, or both. If left untreated, the inflammation can kill the tissue it covers. This killing process is called necrosis. As the tissue dies, the lesion may become infected and begin bleeding. It may also affect more of the surrounding area, as well as the area below the surface. As it deepens, it becomes more crater-like, eventually turning into a festering open wound. Such ulcerations are common on the legs of advanced diabetes patients.

A peptic ulcer is a lesion or chronic open sore on the lining of the stomach or duodenum (the first portion of the small intestine). Normally, a thin, gel-like layer of mucus protects the lining of the stomach and duodenum from gastric acid—hydrochloric acid and pepsinogen, two caustic substances necessary for digestion. But if this layer of mucus is eroded, the underlying tissue is exposed and may become inflamed. If this inflammation is persistent and does not heal, an ulcer may develop. An ulcer sore looks like the top of a volcano. In the center is the crater forming a hole in the stomach lining or duodenal lining. Around the crater is swollen, inflamed tissue.

Scientists used to think that ulcers were caused by too much gastric acid in the stomach and duodenum. They now believe that a failure on the part of the stomach to maintain its mucosal protection, and a bacterium called *Helicobacter pylori*—*H. pylori* for short— are primarily to blame. *H. pylori* bacteria infect the stomach or duodenal lining and cause an ulcer sore in much the same way that bacteria can infect and cause a sore on the skin. The stomach's mucosal protection is eroded by taking aspirin and other nonsteroidal anti-inflammatory drugs, by diet, by stress, and by a variety of other factors. In the next three chapters, we'll examine the causes of peptic ulcer disease in some greater detail.

The symptoms of an ulcer are sometimes hard to read because peptic ulcer disease has many symptoms in common with other diseases. Nausea, heartburn, belching, bloating, and gas are symptoms, but they are also symptoms of dyspepsia and indigestion. A sharp, constant pain between the base of the breastbone and the navel is the classic symptom of a stomach ulcer, but not everyone who gets an ulcer experiences pain in this area.

Eating often relieves ulcer pain because food buffers the lining of the stomach and prevents it from being scalded by gastric acid, however, in another Catch-22, some kinds of food (namely dairy products) increase the production of stomach acid and actually cause more pain in the long run. People with duodenal ulcers feel sharp pain one to three hours after eating. The surest, most ominous signs of an ulcer are blood in the stool or vomit. These are signs of an acute bleeding ulcer. Unfortunately, bleeding is sometimes the first symptom that patients whose ulcers are caused by NSAIDs experience. Chapter 5 looks at ulcer symptoms in detail.

To treat ulcers, doctors often rely on antibiotics, drugs, drug combinations, and supplements. Patients take antibiotics to treat ulcers caused by *H. pylori* bacterial infections. To decrease the amount of acid in the stomach and give ulcers a chance to heal, doctors prescribe H$_2$-blocking drugs and proton pump inhibitors (PPIs). Other drugs fortify the mucosal layer of the stomach to protect the stomach against scalding by gastric acid. These drugs include sucralfate, prostaglandin analogs, and bismuth. As Chapter 8 explains, the supplement Zinc-Carnosine also does a remarkable job of building the stomach's gel-like protective layer of mucus.

With the proper treatment, most peptic ulcers heal in one to three months. In some cases, however, ulcers fail to heal, and this happens for a number of reasons. An ulcer treatment requires taking many pills and tablets. Some patients are delinquent about taking their medication or they abandon their treatment before it is complete. A treatment with antibiotics for an *H. pylori*-caused ulcer cannot succeed if the *H. pylori* strain is resistant to antibiotics.

As I explain in Chapter 6, some strains of *H. pylori* are resistant. Taking non-steroidal anti-inflammatory drugs (NSAIDs) during treatment is another reason why ulcers fail to heal. And as you shall see, these drugs actually cause ulcers. Some people take NSAIDs during treatment without knowing it; others must continue to take NSAIDs during their treatment to relieve osteoporosis or arthritis pain. Of course, many patients discontinue their treatment because they experience too many uncomfortable side effects from the drugs that are meant to help them.

GASTRIC (STOMACH) AND DUODENAL ULCERS

Gastric ulcers occur in the stomach; duodenal ulcers occur in the duodenum (the first portion of the small intestine), most often in the duodenal bulb—the first part of the duodenum that connects it to the stomach. When they are spoken of together, these two types of ulcer are called *peptic ulcers*. In medical terminology, "peptic" refers to a part of the body where digestion takes place and acid is present. A stomach ulcer and gastric ulcer are one and the same. Figure 1.1 shows a diagram of the esophagus, stomach, and duodenum.

Although doctors regard them as different diseases, gastric and duodenal ulcers are for the most part diagnosed and treated the same way. The same factors cause gastric and duodenal ulcers. Both ulcers can cause dyspepsia, a pain or uncomfortable feeling in the pit of the stomach. Gastric and duodenal ulcers differ in a handful of ways:

• About 70 percent of people with gastric ulcers are infected by the *Helicobacter pylori* bacterium; 90 percent of people with duodenal ulcers are also so infected (*H. pylori* is the subject of Chapter 2).

• More gastric ulcers than duodenal ulcers are caused by the use of non-steroidal anti-inflammatory drugs, or NSAIDs (NSAIDs are the subject of Chapter 3).

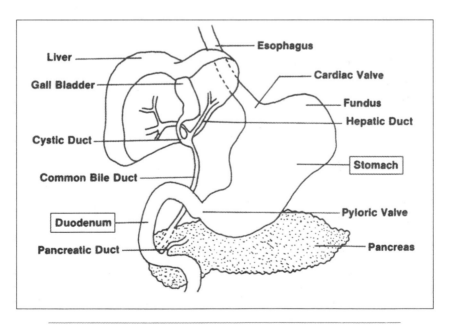

FIGURE 1.1. THE STOMACH AND DUODENUM.

- Gastric ulcers afflict men and women at the same rate, but men get duodenal ulcers twice as often as women.

- People with duodenal ulcers are more likely to secrete ABO blood group antigens in their saliva and have a blood type of O.

If your doctor tells you that you have a peptic ulcer, be sure to ask which type of ulcer you have. This way, you can better understand what your treatment options are.

COMPLICATIONS OF ULCERS

The majority of ulcers heal without difficulty, but an ulcer that goes untreated or fails to heal can become a very serious matter. Ten to twenty percent of patients (far too many) suffer tremendously and, at times, die from ulcer complications. These complications include hemorrhaging, perforation, penetration, and obstruction. These problems can occur without any warning— especially in the case of patients who are taking NSAIDs—as the very first sign or symptom of an ulcer, often in the middle of the night.

Hemorrhage

The lining of the stomach is laced with arteries large and small. How much an ulcer bleeds is largely a matter of chance. If the ulcer sore occurs on top of an important artery, the chances of it bleeding are significant. A mild hemorrhage will leak blood slowly and cause the patient to feel dizzy and lightheaded. A severe hemorrhage will cause the patient to vomit blood and have tar-like, bloody stools. Doctors may stop the bleeding by cauterizing the wound with an endoscope. Most patients who hemorrhage are past the age of 60 and taking NSAIDs. Hemorrhaging occurs in 15 percent of ulcer patients.

Perforation

Perforation occurs when an ulcer sore burrows deep into the wall of the stomach or duodenum, so that gastric acid and other stomach contents are allowed to leak into the otherwise sterile peritoneum—the membrane that lines the wall of the abdomen and covers the abdominal organs. When the peritoneum is inflamed and infected, patients experience sudden, sharp, severe pain and sometimes go into septic shock. This is a life-threatening condition that requires immediate surgery and antibiotic treatment. Perforation occurs in approximately 7 percent of patients, most of whom are women over the age 60. The mortality rate is roughly 19 percent.

Penetration

Penetration occurs when an ulcer sore penetrates the muscular wall of the stomach or, more frequently, the duodenum, and continues into a nearby organ such as the pancreas or liver. The patient experiences sharp, piercing pain in the organ being affected. This condition is treated with antibiotics and sometimes surgery.

Obstruction

An obstruction may occur when an ulcer scar, swelling from inflamed tissue, or an ulcer sore blocks the passage from the stomach to the duodenum. The symptoms of this complication are bloating, lack of appetite, weight loss, and sometimes vomiting. Doctors treat obstructions caused by ulcers by treating the ulcer itself. Sometimes surgery is necessary to treat obstructions caused by scar tissue.

A SHORT HISTORY OF ULCER TREATMENTS

To better understand where science stands today in the treatment of ulcers, we might look back in time to see how far we've come. Peptic disease is probably as old as humanity. Although the Bible doesn't mention it, the first man, Adam, may well have acquired a stress-induced stomach ulcer after he was cast out of the Garden of Eden. Primitive cave dwellers almost certainly suffered from indigestion. They lacked refrigerators. When they were fortunate enough to chase down and kill a fatty, protein-rich animal, they had to devour the entire beast quickly before the meat spoiled. The after-dinner gas in the back of the cave must have been dreadful. Early humans—partially through instinct, experimentation, and

some luck—may have relieved their stomach pain by eating naturally occurring chalk. This substance, known to science as calcium
carbonate, is the primary ingredient in Tums and a handful of
other antacid tablets.

As a testimony to how common dyspepsia and ulcers were and
are, the fact is that nearly every culture has had a folk remedy for
them. These remedies include yellow root tea, chamomile tea (is
there anything chamomile won't cure?), unripe plantain bananas,
sea cucumber, dill, cabbage, ginger root, turmeric, apple cider
vinegar, and licorice (I discuss some ulcer folk remedies in Chapter 7). The Greek physician Diocles of Carystos recorded the first
description of heartburn in 350 B.C.E. The Greeks invented the term
dyspepsia, from *dys*, meaning "bad," and *peptein*, meaning "digestion." Galen (129–210 C.E.), the Roman father of western medicine
who wrote a treatise on dyspepsia, was the first to make the con-

Alexis St. Martin

In 1822, the study of stomach physiology took a leap forward in the
person of Alexis St. Martin, one of the greatest human guinea pigs in
history. St. Martin was a French-Canadian fur trader. During a visit to
Mackinac Island, Michigan—an outpost of the United States Army—he
was shot accidentally in the abdomen and treated by the Army
surgeon on hand, Dr. William Beaumont.

The wound formed a gastric fistula, a hole in the stomach wall the
size of a man's fist. "The man cannot live thirty-six hours; I will come and
see him by and by," Dr. Beaumont told an assistant. For two weeks, all
food that St. Martin ate passed out of the wound in his stomach, and
then, miraculously, his stomach and bowels began functioning normally in spite of the wound. Within a year, under the care of Dr. Beaumont,
the fur trader was as good as new. The only difference between St. Martin and a normal man was the fistula in his stomach, which permitted
Dr. Beaumont to observe the workings of the stomach. "This case affords
a most excellent opportunity of experimenting upon the gastric fluids,
and the process of digestion," Dr. Beaumont reported in the *American
Medical Recorder* in 1825.

nection between tar-like black stools and bleeding in the gastrointestinal tract.

The First Studies

Medical science, beholden to the ancient Greeks and Romans, took a long nap during the Middle Ages and Renaissance. Not until the lifting of the prohibition against autopsies and dissections in the eighteenth century did physicians learn more about ulcers and the workings of the gastrointestinal tract. In 1727, the Englishman Christopher Rawlinson wrote the fist clinical description of a perforated ulcer. Scientists understood that gastric juices played a role in digestion, but they believed that the juices were merely swallowed saliva. Advances in surgery permitted German and English physicians to operate on perforated ulcers in the late 1800s. The discovery of X-rays by Wilhelm Conrad Roentgen in 1895 allowed

For ten years, occasionally dangling food tied to a string into his subject's stomach, Dr. Beaumont conducted some 230 experiments on the action of the stomach and saw firsthand the role of acid in digestion. Dr. Beaumont was the first to identify the hydrochloric acid in gastric juice. He understood hydrochloric acid's antibacterial function and its role in digestion. His book, *Experiments and Observations on the Gastric Juice and the Physiology of Digestion,* published in 1833, revolutionized medical thinking about digestion and brought glory to the American medical establishment.

The story of Dr. Beaumont, the stern Yankee from New England, and his patient Alexis St. Martin, the rugged fur trader from the wilds of Canada, is remembered today not only because it advanced medical science, but because it raises intriguing questions with regard to medical ethics. Dr. Beaumont could have closed the wound in St. Martin's abdomen. However, he left it open so he could conduct experiments. Although his experiments proved extremely useful for medical science, did Dr. Beaumont have the right to treat Alexis St. Martin as he did?

Whatever you think of Dr. Beaumont's ethics, you will be glad to know that Alexis St. Martin lived to a ripe old age in spite of his stomach wound. He died at age 84 in 1880.

physicians to diagnose ulcers, however crudely, without having to open up the stomach.

The Modern Era

In the middle of the twentieth century, the treatment of ulcers entered what I consider a dark period, when physicians decided that surgery was the best way to treat ulcers. Removing the ulcerous part of the stomach, removing the duodenum, and in some instances removing the stomach altogether were considered valid ulcer treatments. Unfortunately, patients had to be hospitalized for long periods of time after these procedures. Many found themselves after surgery with inert, dysfunctional stomachs that were not capable of digesting food properly. Patients' quality of life suffered accordingly.

Starting around 1940, medical science began to understand that gastric acid plays an essential role in ulcer formation. The doctors of the day counseled their patients to avoid stress as a means of curing ulcer disease. This notion that stress is the primary cause of ulcer disease persists today. Patients took to their beds and ate a bland diet of oatmeal and malted milk to lower stomach acidity. In the 1960s and 1970s, doctors subscribed to the idea of an "ulcer personality," an aggressive go-getter type who was more prone to peptic ulcer disease.

Previous to 1972, patients took antacid tablets and bismuth (known to us as Pepto-Bismol) to lower their stomach acidity, but 1972 saw the advent of a new kind of drug called H_2-blockers that worked wonders by lowering the production of stomach acid and relieving ulcer pain. In the 1980s, drugs called proton pump inhibitors, which reduced acid production even more effectively, became available. Meanwhile, the Australian scientists Barry Marshall and Robin Warren made a remarkable discovery that turned the current thinking about ulcer disease on its ear. They determined that a bacterium called *Helicobacter pylori (H. pylori)* was responsible for the majority of cases of peptic ulcer disease. As I explain in Chapter 2, persuading the medical community at large to treat ulcers by eradicating *H. pylori* was an uphill battle that lasted ten years. But, by 1990, treating the bacterium that causes ulcers with antibiotics became a standard anti-ulcer therapy.

Looking Toward Natural Treatments

In keeping with the notion that the best medicine is preventative medicine, some doctors are recommending natural supplements to guard against and treat ulcers. Zinc-Carnosine is one such natural supplement. Instead of interfering with the stomach's production of gastric acid, Zinc-Carnosine soothes ulcers by strengthening the stomach's natural defenses. In other words, it helps the stomach do what the stomach wants to do successfully on its own.

Because digestion is a continuum, a long process that begins with the salivary glands and ends in the colon, interfering with the natural digestive process in one area always has consequences further down. Halting the production of digestive acids in the stomach, for example, allows bacteria and toxins that would normally be killed by digestive acids to enter the small and large intestines. This can have negative health consequences. Zinc-Carnosine, however, does not interfere with gastric acid production. The supplement acts as a buffer to strengthen the mucosal layer that protects the stomach from scalding by gastric acid. It heals ulcers, but still allows for the natural process of digestion to occur.

CONCLUSION

The treatment of peptic ulcer disease has come a long way. A half century ago, at best, someone with a peptic ulcer was made to eat a bland diet of malted milk and oatmeal; at worst, this person went under the knife and had all or part of his or her stomach removed. Now the majority of ulcers can be treated successfully with drugs and drug combinations that reduce gastric acid production and kill *H. pylori,* the recently discovered bacterium that can cause peptic ulcers.

While it's true that the number of people who get peptic ulcers has dropped since the 1970s thanks to better treatments, doctors are bracing themselves for a rise in the incidence of peptic ulcer disease. NSAIDs cause ulcers, and their use is at an all time high—and likely to get higher as baby boomers enter their retirement years. The elderly have to take NSAIDs for osteoporosis and other age-related diseases. For this reason, it is essential to find new treatments, and natural supplements such as Zinc-Carnosine may be the answer for many patients, as it does a wonderful job of protecting the stomach lining against scalding by gastric acid—without disrupting the natural digestive process.

Outside the United States and the rest of the industrialized world, the chief culprit in peptic ulcer disease is not NSAIDs, but the *H. pylori* bacterium. The next chapter looks at this bacterium, explains how it damages the stomach and duodenum, and shows how it is spread—among other issues.

2

Helicobacter Pylori

elicobacter pylori (H. pylori) is a bacterium, or microorganism, that causes gastritis and peptic ulcers—in other words, stomach ulcers and ulcers that occur in the duodenum (the first portion of the small intestine). Half of the world's population is infected with *H. pylori* bacteria, arguably the most ever-present bacterium on the planet. *H. pylori* is to blame for roughly 75 percent of stomach ulcers and 90 percent of duodenal ulcers, yet the vast majority of infected people do not get an ulcer or any other gastrointestinal disease.

This chapter examines the mysterious *H. pylori* bacterium. I recount how the bacterium was discovered in 1983 and how this discovery changed the way that ulcers are understood and treated. I explain how the bacterium is spread, how it survives in the harsh acidic environment of the stomach, and how *H. pylori* infections are diagnosed. This chapter looks beyond gastric and duodenal ulcers, to other diseases that may or may not be caused by an *H. pylori* infection. Finally, I explore what may be called a heretical view—why being infected by *H. pylori* might actually have health advantages.

WHAT ARE BACTERIA?

A bacterium is a living, microscopic, single-celled organism. All bacteria are capable of reproducing, usually very quickly. Bacterial cells are much smaller and simpler than human cells. They consist of an outer cell membrane that houses the cytoplasm, enzymes, and amino acids that the cell produces to survive. In the center, there is a tightly wound ball of DNA.

At any given time, your gastrointestinal tract harbors three to four pounds of bacteria, most of it in the colon. There are ten times as many bacterial cells in your digestive tract than there are cells in the rest of your body. If this fact alarms you, you will be glad to know that most of these bacteria are actually good for your health. In the digestive tract, healthy bacteria such as lactobacilli and bifidobacteria fight off and kill harmful bacteria such as *E. coli*. In effect, these beneficial bacteria act as antibiotics because they kill off cells that can cause disease and cancer.

H. pylori is one kind of bacterial cell that can survive in the human body. As I explain in this chapter, *H. pylori* has evolved into an organism that is capable of surviving in the harsh acidic environment of the stomach. Doctors treat *H. pylori* infections with antibiotics. One of the major drawbacks of this treatment is that antibiotics kill beneficial bacteria in the digestive tract as well as *H. pylori* and other dangerous bacteria. Moreover, the use of antibiotics may produce hardier, antibiotic-resistant strains of *H. pylori.*

DISCOVERY OF *H. PYLORI*

The discovery of *H. pylori* bacteria in 1983 forever changed the way that ulcers are understood and treated. Prior to this discovery by Australian scientists Barry Marshall and Robin Warren, physicians believed that excessive production of acid in the stomach caused ulcers. To lower the production of stomach acid and relieve ulcer pain, physicians had their patients renounce spicy food, alcohol, caffeine, and other foods that were supposed to encourage the production of stomach acid. "No acid, no ulcer," was the byword. Patients ate a diet of bland foods, dairy products, and malted milk. Because stress was supposed to cause ulcers, ulcer patients were told to get plenty of bed rest and avoid stressful situations. In the case of hemorrhaging ulcers and perforations, doctors sometimes treated the patients by removing part of the stomach.

Sighting the Spiral-Shaped Bacteria

The idea that a bacterium could cause disease was not foreign to physicians. Thanks to the efforts of pioneering bacteriologist Dr. Robert Koch and others, physicians understood as early as the 1890s that bacteria cause tuberculosis, but they simply couldn't conceive of bacteria causing a peptic ulcer. How could bacteria survive in the caustic, highly acidic human stomach? Wouldn't the bacteria die before they could cause an infection? One hundred years ago, German scientists doing postmortem biopsies of patients who had died of stomach ulcers were the first to notice *H. pylori* bacteria (see Figure 2.1 below). They decided, however, that the unusual, spiral-shaped bacteria they saw in their microscopes grew on the tissue samples as a result of contamination in the laboratory. No bacteria could survive in the stomach's acidic environment. The German scientists tried but failed to grow the bacteria in a culture, and over time their findings were lost to obscurity.

In 1979, picking up where the German scientists left off a century before, Robin Warren, a pathologist working at the Royal Perth Hospital in Western Australia, also noticed unusual spiral-shaped bacteria in stomach biopsy tissue samples. The bacteria intrigued him for several reasons. They appeared in biopsy samples that showed signs of inflammation, but not in other samples. Where the bacteria appeared in greater numbers, inflammation

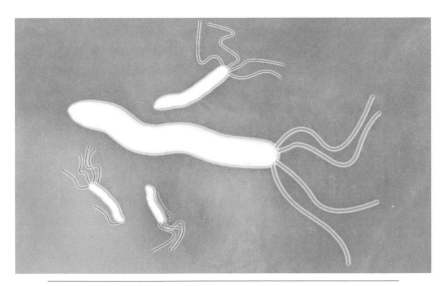

FIGURE 2.1. *H. PYLORI* BACTERIA.

was greater. Curiously, the bacteria had managed to work their way underneath the stomach's thick, gel-like mucus layer, which protects the stomach from hydrochloric acid. These conspicuous bacteria, Warren decided, may have something to do with inflaming the stomach tissue and causing ulcers.

Isolating the Bacteria

The next step was to isolate the bacteria for study. With the help of Barry J. Marshall, a trainee in internal medicine, Warren tried with no success to culture bacterial samples from three dozen patients. *H. pylori* is a temperamental, slow-growing bacterium. The two scientists might never have cultured *H. pylori* had not serendipity worked in their favor. To celebrate Easter, Warren and Marshall took an extended holiday in April of 1982, and, doing so, they left *H. pylori* samples in the incubator for five days rather than the usual two. When the two scientists returned from their Easter holiday, they discovered *H. pylori* colonies growing successfully in the culture dish. The bacteria, it turned out, needed more time to grow in the laboratory than other bacteria common to the gastrointestinal tract.

Because the bacterium resembled *Campylobacter,* a bacterium known to cause enteritis, a disease of the small intestine, Warren and Marshall initially named their discovery *Campylobacter pylori.* Both men were convinced that the bacterium caused gastritis and stomach ulcers. They conducted a study—later published in the British journal *Lancet*—of one hundred people undergoing endoscopy, in which the researchers concluded that 100 percent of people with duodenal ulcers and 80 percent of people with stomach ulcers were infected with *H. pylori.* (Ulcers in the remaining patients were attributed to the use of non-steroidal anti-inflammatory drugs, or NSAIDs, a known cause of stomach ulcers.) In another experiment, Marshall demonstrated how bismuth, a common treatment for ulcers, could kill *H. pylori* in a petri dish. He gave bismuth to his ulcer patients at Fremantle Hospital, but they did not appear to gain any benefit from chewing the bismuth tablets. Some showed improvement, but all relapsed. Why did bismuth kill *H. pylori* in the petri dish but not in the stomachs of his ulcer patients?

Convincing the Medical Community

In September 1983, Marshall presented the findings on *Campy-lobacter* infections at the International Workshop in Brussels, and they were greeted with scorn and dismay. The notion that a bacterium could cause ulcers was unthinkable. Martin Blaser, then of the Vanderbilt University School of Medicine, thought it was "the most preposterous thing I'd ever heard; I thought, 'This guy is a madman.'" Dr. Blaser has since become a leading researcher of *H. pylori* and an eloquent interpreter of how the bacterium lives and grows. Another scientist at the conference, Dr. David Forman of the Imperial Cancer Research Fund, called the claim by Marshall and Warren a "totally crazy hypothesis."

The totally crazy hypothesis was rejected not only because it was so new and seemingly implausible, but also because the Australians had not succeeded in proving a cause-and-effect relationship between *H. pylori* infection and stomach ulcers. The theory was that instead of the bacteria causing inflammation to the lining of the stomach, the bacteria opportunistically sought out inflamed tissue. In other words, *H. pylori* was an opportunistic bacterium that came after stomach inflammation, not before it.

"Those were frustrating times for me," Barry Marshall said of those years. "Most of the experts believed that the presence of *H. pylori* in those who turned up with ulcer problems was just a coincidence. I planned to give myself an ulcer, then treat myself, to prove that *H. pylori* can be a pathogen in normal people. I thought about it for a few weeks, then decided to just do it. Luckily, I only developed a temporary infection."

The normal procedure would have been to infect animals with *H. pylori* to see if they developed stomach or duodenal ulcers, but animals, it was thought at the time, were immune to *H. pylori* infections (since then, *Helicobacter* bacteria have been found in primates, dogs, cats, and rodents). Because he couldn't experiment with animals, Barry Marshall decided that his only recourse was to use himself as a guinea pig. In 1984, after an endoscopy determined that he had no *H. pylori* bacteria in his stomach, Marshall prepared an *H. pylori* broth and drank it. Five days later, he experienced abdominal pain, vomiting, and nausea, the characteristic symptoms of gastritis.

An endoscopy and microscopy showed that spiral-shaped *H. pylori* bacteria had indeed established themselves in Marshall's stomach. Much to his pleasure—insofar as anybody with gastritis can experience pleasure—Marshall had succeeded in infecting himself and proving that *H. pylori* causes gastritis. He took an antibiotic and was soon cured. While his experiment proved that *H. pylori* causes gastritis, it didn't prove that the bacterium causes ulcers. Marshall had cured himself with antibiotics before an ulcer could develop in his stomach.

By now, RNA sequencing and examinations of the bacterium using electron microscopes had made it clear that the newly isolated bacteria did not belong to the genus *Campylobacter* after all. A new name, *Helicobacter pylori*, was chosen. The genus name *Helicobacter* was selected because of the bacterium's helical, or spiral, shape. The species name *pylori* was chosen because ulcers often appear close to the pyloric valve—the sphincter muscle that separates the stomach from the duodenum.

Initial Studies

Starting in 1985, Marshall undertook a two-year, double-blind study of one hundred patients with duodenal ulcers who also had *H. pylori* infections. The object of this study was to find out if eradicating *H. pylori* in these patients healed their duodenal ulcers. The study involved a placebo and three medicines: the H_2-blocker cimetidine (Tagamet), the common ulcer medicine bismuth, and the antibiotic tinidazole (chemically, this antibiotic is similar to Flagyl). H_2 blockers are medicines designed to reduce acid production in the stomach.

Patients were randomly separated into four groups and took the medicines and the placebo as follows:

- Group 1 took the H_2 blocker and the antibiotic.

- Group 2 took the H_2 blocker and a placebo.

- Group 3 took bismuth and the antibiotic.

- Group 4 took bismuth and a placebo.

By far, the most effective therapy was the bismuth-antibiotic combination taken by Group 3. In that group, twenty of the twenty-seven subjects no longer had *H. pylori* infections. After ten weeks, all patients were examined by endoscopy. Ninety-two percent of patients who no longer had *H. pylori* in their gastrointestinal tracts had been cured of their duodenal ulcers. However, in the case of patients who still harbored the bacteria, only 61 percent were cured. Marshall and his colleagues wrote about their study, "Our results imply that *C. pylori [H. pylori]* is the most important aetiologic factor so far described for duodenal ulcer." They had shown an indisputable link between *H. pylori* and ulcers. Just as important, they had shown that taking a bismuth-antibiotic combination is the most effective way to treat ulcers. Today, more than two decades after Marshall's original study, treating patients with a combination of antibiotics and bismuth, along with an H_2-blocking drug such as ranitidine (Zantac), is the standard ulcer treatment. (Chapter 6 explains drug therapies for peptic ulcer disease.)

Acceptance

As news of Marshall and Warren's work spread through the medical community, other research groups took up the task of examining the role of *H. pylori* in gastritis and ulcers. Between 1988 and 1993, no less than 1,191 scientific papers about *H. pylori* and peptic ulcer disease appeared in medical journals and magazines. In a landmark 1986 experiment, David Graham of Baylor College of Medicine conducted the first randomized study of antibiotic therapy for the treatment of ulcers in the United States. As Marshall had done a year before, Graham used a combination of antibiotics and an H_2 blocker to successfully treat ulcer patients. The study was published in the prestigious *Annals of Internal Medicine*. Warren and Marshall's theory about *H. pylori* and peptic ulcers had ceased being a theory and had become an accepted fact.

In 1994, a Consensus Development Conference sponsored by The National Institutes of Health (NIH) concluded that there is indeed a strong association between *H. pylori* and peptic ulcers. The NIH recommended treating *H. pylori*-infected ulcer patients with a combination of antibiotics to kill the ulcer-causing bacteria and secretion-stopping (anti-secretory) drugs to lower inflammation and ulcer pain.

HOW WIDESPREAD IS *H. PYLORI*?

When you are exposed to a bacterium, your body produces anti-bodies so that next time you're exposed, the antibodies can fight and eradicate the bacterial invader. Because the body produces antibodies for all bacteria, including *H. pylori*, physicians can deter-mine who has been infected by *H. pylori* simply by testing blood for the presence of *H. pylori* antibodies. By studying blood samples that have been stored in clinics and blood banks, researchers can see how prevalent the bacteria are in different sample groups. They can even examine frozen blood samples taken years before to see how *H. pylori* infection rates from years past compare to infection rates today.

After modern medicine became convinced that *H. pylori* causes gastritis and ulcers, researchers studied many frozen blood sam-ples. Using the data along with present-day findings, researchers discovered that *H. pylori* bacteria may be one of the most ubiquitous bacteria on the planet. By some estimates, 3 billion people—or half the world's population—have been infected. The bacteria are found in every country, but are easier to acquire where people live under crowded conditions and sanitary standards are lax.

The following statistics give a picture of how prevalent *H. pylori* infections are in the United States:

- About 50 percent of Americans are infected with *H. pylori* bacteria by age 60. Approximately 20 percent of people under age 40 are infected. People born before 1950 are twice as likely to be infected.

- People in higher socio-economic brackets—those with higher incomes and levels of education—tend to be infected with *H. pylori* less than those in lower brackets.

- *H. pylori* infections are fairly uncommon among children; however, the bacteria is often acquired and harbored in early childhood.

- The infection rates tend to be highest in communities with immi-grant populations.

- Since 1968, there has been a 50 percent decline in the number of Americans who are infected.

The statistics just given are typical of the United States as well as other industrialized countries, but the picture in developing countries is considerably bleaker:

- About 70 percent of children are infected by age 10.

- Infection rates vary from 70 to 90 percent.

The large number of children in developing countries who are being infected by *H. pylori* is particularly troubling because some researchers believe that infections acquired in childhood are more likely to cause gastritis, peptic ulcers, and stomach cancer. The belief is that the bacteria have more time in which to damage stomach tissue if the bacteria are acquired early in life. We are likely to see high rates of stomach and duodenal ulcers in the developing world in the years to come.

In both industrialized and developing countries, most people are exposed to the *H. pylori* bacteria within the first ten years of life. Most people who are infected acquire the bacterium when they are children, although the infection may not lead to an ulcer until adulthood. In several studies, researchers were able to examine, in the same subjects, frozen blood samples taken over a period of many years to gauge the rate at which people pick up *H. pylori* infections as they grow older. As I explained earlier, researchers can tell who has been infected by testing blood for the presence of *H. pylori* antibodies. In general, the studies showed that adults acquire *H. pylori* quite slowly, if at all, and that most infections occur in childhood.

In one Australian study, for example, researchers compared blood samples from 20 to 40 year olds that were taken between the years 1967 and 1970 to samples that were taken from the same subjects in 1978, and then again in 1990. In samples from the 1967 to 1970 period, 38 percent of the subjects had *H. pylori* antibodies; the 1978 samples showed 40.9 percent had the antibodies; and in the 1990 samples, antibodies were present in 34.8 percent. The number of those infected actually shrank between 1978 and 1990. This study and others like it indicated that most *H. pylori* infections occur during childhood.

In an interesting study conducted in Texas, researchers

attempted to pinpoint the age at which children are infected. The study made use of blood samples taken at three-year intervals from 224 children between the years 1975 and 1996 (the samples were taken originally to examine the risk factors of heart disease). By 1996, the twenty-first year of the study, 24.5 percent of the children had been infected by *H. pylori*. What follows is the children's yearly rate of infection:

- **Age 1 to 3.** This first blood sample taken at the start of the study showed that 8 percent of the children were infected.

- **Age 4 to 6.** This sampling showed 2.1 percent were infected each year—the highest yearly rate of infection in the study.

- **Age 7 to 9.** These samples showed 1.5 percent were infected each year.

The annual infection rate continued to drop until it reached 0.3 percent at year 21. It appears from this study that strategies for preventing the spread of *H. pylori* bacteria should be aimed at children in the under-10 age group, especially children in the rambunctious 4 to 6 age bracket. In other words, young kids should wash their hands more carefully. It is extremely important to establish the habit of thorough hand washing every time one uses the restroom.

Keep in mind that harboring *H. pylori* bacteria doesn't mean that you will develop a peptic ulcer or even get gastritis. The majority of people who carry *H. pylori* infections in their stomachs experience no ill effects. I will discuss why this happens later in this chapter.

HOW *H. PYLORI* BACTERIA ARE SPREAD

H. pylori bacteria spread more readily in places where sanitary conditions are poor. This may explain why infection rates are dropping in the United States. Hospitalizations in the United States for gastric ulcers increased beginning in 1900, peaked in 1950, and have been declining ever since. In the first half of the twentieth century, record numbers of Americans moved from the secluded farm to the crowded city, where they acquired *H. pylori* infections in crowded tenements and block housing. But starting in 1950, sanitary conditions improved in the cities, and, moreover, Americans started moving to the relatively cleaner suburbs. Under these better sanitary conditions, fewer children were exposed to *H. pylori*, which may be the reason why, fifty years later, fewer Americans are hospitalized for ulcers.

Still, until science invents a microscopic Sherlock Holmes and a miniscule Dr. Watson, no one can be entirely certain how *H. pylori* or any other bacteria travel from person to person. Nevertheless, scientists have identified several different means by which the *H. pylori* bacterium is spread. They are explained below.

Fecal-Oral Route

H. pylori have been cultured in stool; the bacteria can live in feces. *H. pylori* infections are more likely to occur where sanitary conditions are poor and people live in crowded conditions. Many bacteria are transmitted through the fecal-oral route. Inadequate hand washing between the toilet and the kitchen, eating contaminated food, and mishandling baby diapers are ways in which fecal-oral transmission can occur. In families with many children and in crowded institutions such as orphanages, transmission occurs frequently through this route.

Contaminated Water

DNA consistent with *H. pylori* has been found in the water supply of Peru, where the rate of infection is extremely high. As is the case with many countries lacking a modernized waste removal system, Peru's inadequate sanitary systems account for these rampant rates of infection. Water used for drinking and cooking, as well as foods and eating utensils that are washed in tainted water, are also sources of transmission.

Oral-Oral by Acid Reflux

The bacteria may be spread when people with gastroesophageal reflux disease, or GERD, experience an acid reflux or belch, and the *H. pylori* germs rise from the stomach into the throat and mouth, where they can be transmitted to others. Belching and acid reflux—the rising of gastric juices from the stomach into the esophagus—are symptoms of gastritis, a disease associated with *H. pylori* infection. *H. pylori* has been detected in the dental plaque of people who have been infected with the bacteria.

Insects

One theory holds that the *H. pylori* bacteria can be spread from person to person on the proboscis and legs of the common housefly. To test this theory, researchers at St. Elizabeth's Medical Center in Boston conducted an experiment in which they exposed separate groups of adult houseflies either to *H. pylori* bacteria or to a sterile control plate. Flies exposed to *H. pylori* were tested at six-hour intervals for the presence of the bacteria. The researchers discovered that the bacteria remained on their bodies for up to twelve hours; it remained in their intestinal tracts for up to thirty hours. No bacteria were found on the control group.

Houseflies hatch and feed on excrement. The fine hairs on the insect's proboscis are perfectly suited for collecting bacteria. The insect's six legs secrete a sticky substance that is ideal for picking up pathogens. It is easy to see how flies might harbor *H. pylori* and spread it to the food that humans eat. However, the St. Elizabeth's Medical Center researchers caution that it is too early to say for certain whether houseflies really do transmit *H. pylori* bacteria.

DISEASES ASSOCIATED WITH *H. PYLORI* INFECTION

Infection by *H. pylori* has been implicated in a host of diseases, not just stomach ulcers and duodenal ulcers. In the next few pages, I look at these diseases and focus primarily on gastritis and stomach cancer.

H. Pylori and Stomach Cancer

Cancer is a complex disease that can affect any organ or system of the body. Causes of the disease include heredity and cell damage caused by toxins and radiation. Some researchers believe that cancer results when genes that are normally dormant begin helping to produce cancer cells. An infection, pollutant, or other outside agent triggers the genes to start producing cancer cells. In some respects, cancer is a natural occurrence in the body. With approximately 100 million cells dividing in the body per day, some replications are bound to occur in error. According to a recent study, six detectable tumors are produced each year in the body of the average American. If you went to the doctor every day of the year and were probed in the right locations, you would be diagnosed with cancer six times. In most people, however, the immune system eradicates cancerous tumors before they become a health issue.

As cancer cells grow in number, they may bleed, interfere with vital organs, press on nerves, or block arteries. Some cancers—stomach cancer is one of them—are slow growing and may take many years to develop, while other cancers grow quickly. The majority of cancers of the gastrointestinal tract occur in the colon and rectum, probably because foods remain there longer and toxins cannot be expelled as quickly. At 50 thousand deaths per year, colorectal cancer trails only lung cancer as the leading cause of cancer-related death in the United States. By contrast, stomach cancer causes the deaths of about 15 thousand Americans annually. Stomach cancer rates have been dropping in the United States since the 1950s.

After it became known that the *H. pylori* bacterium causes stomach and duodenal ulcers, scientists began looking at whether the bacteria are responsible for stomach cancer as well. Scientists knew that people who have ulcerative colitis, a chronic inflammation of the colon, were inclined to get colon cancer, and they reasoned that a chronic inflammation of the gastric mucosa in the stomach caused by *H. pylori* might similarly bring about stomach cancer. Many studies were done on stomach cancer patients to discover whether they were infected with *H. pylori*. The Eurogast Study Group's findings, published in 1993 in the *Lancet,* were typical: "Our findings are consistent with an approximately six-fold increased risk of gastric cancer in populations with 100-percent *H. pylori* infection compared with populations that have no infection." Studies showed that people infected by *H. pylori* are three to six times more likely to develop stomach cancer.

In 1994, the World Health Organization based in Geneva, Switzerland, declared *H. pylori* a class-1 carcinogen. This rank is reserved for the most dangerous cancer-causing agents. Other class-1 carcinogens include asbestos, arsenic, the hepatitis C virus, mustard gas, plutonium-239, and tobacco smoke.

Still, whether *H. pylori* can be linked definitively to stomach cancer remains very much an open question on account of the "African paradox." In parts of Africa (and India) where rates of *H. pylori* infection are as high as 90 percent and people acquire the bacteria at an early age, stomach cancer rates are equal to or lower than those found in the United States, where only 50 percent of the population is infected with *H. pylori* by age 60. Furthermore, few people in the United States, Africa, and elsewhere who have been infected with *H. pylori* actually develop stomach cancer. It is very likely that other factors besides *H. pylori* infection—diet, a family history of stomach ulcers—play a role in whether a person gets stomach cancer. Consumption of smoked fish, salty food, and alcohol are also believed to be contributors. Chapter 4 looks into the causes of peptic ulcers apart from *H. pylori* infection and NSAID use.

H. Pylori and Gastritis

Gastritis is not a disease per se but an inflammation of the stomach lining. The most common symptoms are abdominal pain, excessive belching, nausea, abdominal bloating, and a burning feeling in the upper abdomen. The inflammation is caused by white blood cells that move into the lining of the stomach as a result of infection or injury. Gastritis almost always precedes an ulcer. Over time, gastritis can also cause the lesions that precede cancer.

Infection by *H. pylori* bacteria and the long-term use of NSAIDs are the primary causes of gastritis, with the *H. pylori* bacterium mainly to blame. In the stomach, *H. pylori* bacteria emit urease and other toxins, and white blood cells assemble at the site of the infection to fight these invaders. This infiltration of white blood cells, however, can cause uncomfortable swelling and inflammation in much the same way that an infiltration of white blood cells causes a sprained wrist or an ankle to swell. This uncomfortable swelling in the stomach causes gastritis.

In the past, doctors treated gastritis by prescribing medicine to reduce stomach acid and thereby relieve symptoms. However, to treat chronic cases of gastritis, doctors now prescribe an antibiotic treatment. The reasoning is to cure the *H. pylori* infection that caused the gastritis.

Other Diseases Associated with *H. Pylori*

Besides stomach ulcers, duodenal ulcers, stomach cancer, and gastritis, *H. pylori* bacteria have been implicated in several other diseases, which are explained below.

Gastric Lymphoma

Gastric lymphoma tumors, like *H. pylori* infections, tend to appear in the antrum, the lower part of the stomach. Some researchers believe that the presence of *H. pylori* and tumors in the same location indicates that *H. pylori* may be responsible for the tumors. Moreover, curing *H. pylori* tends to make these tumors regress.

Nonulcerative Dyspepsia

Nonulcerative dyspepsia is the catchall term for an assortment of symptoms—nausea, bloating, burning pain in the upper abdominal—not caused by an ulcer. Usually, the patient experiences these painful symptoms shortly after eating and relieves them by taking antacid tablets. People with dyspepsia are more likely to be infected with *H. pylori* than people without the condition.

Sudden Infant Death Syndrome (SIDS)

SIDS is the sudden unexplained death of a baby less than one year old. Scientists from the University of Manchester looked at tissue from the stomachs, lungs, and windpipes of thirty-two infants, age seven months or younger, who had died of SIDS. In twenty-eight of thirty-two tissue samples, researchers found genes that indicated the presence of an *H. pylori* infection.

Hypochlorhydria

Hypochlorhydria is a lack of hydrochloric acid in the stomach. Hydrochloric acid helps with digestion and kills germs as they arrive. As you age, the parietal cells in your stomach lining that produce hydrochloric acid age as well, and become less efficient. According to some reports, half of the people over age 60 have hypochlorhydria. Sufferers of the disease have trouble digesting food and absorbing vitamin B_{12}, a problem that can lead to pernicious anemia. They are also more susceptible to infection from *H. pylori* because their stomachs don't produce enough acid to kill the bacteria. However, whether *H. pylori* contributes to hypochlorhydria, or the deficiency of hydrochloric acid permits *H. pylori* bacteria to thrive, is unknown.

Halitosis

Halitosis is better known as chronic bad breath. Because antibiot-

Germs and Disease

When I was in medical school in the 1950s, my professors would have laughed at the suggestion that a bacterium such as *H. pylori* could cause peptic ulcers or another chronic health problem. But the discovery of *H. pylori* as the cause of peptic ulcers, along with similar discoveries, has given rise to a new school of thought in medical science. This school holds that bacteria and viruses are responsible not just for short-lived illnesses such as colds and flues, but for chronic health problems as well. According to some researchers, many more diseases than we realize are caused by bacterial and viral infections. Germs have been blamed for asthma, arthritis, allergies, heart disease, diabetes, cancer, and even obesity.

Thanks to new testing methods, molecular biologists can examine tissue more closely than before, and they are finding evidence that microbes cause damage above and beyond the initial infection. Some microbes take advantage of the body's immune response and trick the body into attacking healthy tissue. Others, like *H. pylori,* attract an abundance of white blood cells, and, when these cells assemble at the site of the infection, chronic inflammation results. Chronic inflammation has been cited as a cause of heart disease, asthma, and allergies.

Consider the following examples (at right) of bacteria and viruses causing chronic disease:

ic treatments for *H. pylori* have been known to relieve halitosis as well, some argue that *H. pylori* causes bad breath. More likely, the antibiotics that are given to eradicate *H. pylori* also kill the bacteria in the mouth and sinus cavities that cause bad breath.

SURVIVING IN THE GASTRIC SOUP

In the stomach is a scathing gastric soup made of hydrochloric acid and various digestive enzymes whose job is to break down food for the purpose of digestion, and, for the purpose of immunity, to kill anything that might do harm to the body, including viruses and bacteria. To keep the walls of the stomach from being harmed by this gastric acid, your body coats the stomach lining with a pro-

- Infection by hepatitis B or C greatly increases the risk of getting liver cancer.

- The human papilloma virus, the most prevalent sexually transmitted disease, is the culprit in 99 percent of cervical cancers.

- Studies have linked *Chlamydia pneumoniae,* a bacterium, with arteriosclerosis, or hardening of the arteries.

- The adenovirus that causes a strain of the common cold may be responsible for obesity. Studies show that 20 to 30 percent of overweight people are infected with adenovirus-36, while only 5 percent of the lean population is infected.

Writing in *Scientific American,* the noted microbiologist Martin J. Blaser offered this assessment of the microbe school of disease, "I believe that *H. pylori* are very likely the first in a class of slow-acting bacteria that may well account for a number of perplexing diseases that we are facing today." If it turns out to be true that bacteria and viruses are responsible for more diseases than we know, antibiotics, anti-viral drugs, and vaccines will play a larger role in medical treatment in the years ahead. Antioxidants—vitamin C, vitamin E, beta-carotene, and others—might also play a larger role. Antioxidants can repair tissue that has been damaged by bacteria and viruses. Prunes, raisins, blueberries, and blackberries are among the best natural sources of antioxidants.

tective gel-like layer of mucus. (Zinc-Carnosine helps prevent ulcers by strengthening this mucus layer.) *H. pylori* can evade immune-system defenses by hiding in the stomach's mucus layer. Wily, tenacious, and stubborn, this bacteria has defense mechanisms for withstanding attacks by the gastric acid and white blood cells that are present in the stomach. A recent study conducted at the New York University School of Medicine showed that humans have been carrying the *H. pylori* bacterium for at least 11,000 years, and that migrating Asians brought it to the New World long before Europeans arrived there. The bacterium has lived successfully inside humans for a long time.

In a typical *H. pylori* infection, four-fifths of the bacterial colonies inhabit the mucus-secreting epithelial cells, and the other fifth attaches itself to the stomach lining, called the gastric epithelium. The 5-percent oxygen level in the stomach's mucus layer is ideal for *H. pylori* bacteria. The microorganism's spiral shape and four to seven flagellae, or "tails," permit it to be highly mobile. The bacterium can burrow into the stomach's mucus layer and avoid destruction by gastric acid and white blood cells. When the stomach contracts to push its contents into the small intestine, *H. pylori* bacteria can swim upstream (so to speak) and avoid being expelled. Karen Ottemann of the University of California at Santa Cruz has done some interesting research to show that *H. pylori* bacteria don't move at random through the mucosal layer, but actually target weak areas that are more susceptible to infection. *H. pylori* does this by means of chemoreceptors—proteins on the bacteria's membrane surface that are capable of sensing where an infection is likely to succeed.

Unless it is treated with antibiotics, an *H. pylori* infection usually lasts for a lifetime. Many factors contribute to the bacteria's survival, and are detailed below.

Neutralizes Gastric Acid

H. pylori bacterial cells are able to neutralize gastric acid and create an alkaline microenvironment in which they can flourish. *H. pylori* neutralize gastric acid by emitting an enzyme called urease. An enzyme is a protein that cells produce to carry out certain actions. This enzyme acts upon urea, a substance found in saliva and the stomach's gastric juices, to create ammonia and carbon dioxide. These two chemicals, combined with water in the stomach, produce ammonium bicarbonate, an alkaline substance capable of neutralizing gastric acid. In effect, *H. pylori* bacterial cells insulate themselves from the stomach's harsh acidic environment by emitting urease. One way that doctors test for the presence of *H. pylori* is to administer a urea breath test, which is used to detect urease, the enzyme produced by *H. pylori*.

Hides in the Stomach Mucosa

The layer of mucus that protects the stomach lining from hydrochloric acid also serves as a hiding place for *H. pylori* bacteria. Because many of the white blood cells that normally fight bacterial infections are too large to penetrate the mucosal layer, *H. pylori* bacteria are safe from these white blood cells. Many physicians treat their patients with high concentrations of antibiotics because they believe that only these high dosages can infiltrate the mucosal layer and eradicate *H. pylori*. As I explain in Chapter 6, I disagree with this aggressive antibiotic treatment.

Takes Advantage of White Blood Cells

H. pylori may actually hijack the stomach's defense system to make it work in the bacteria's favor. When an infection occurs, the stomach produces a sugar molecule called sLex (sialyl-di-Lewis) that signals white blood cells to hurry to the scene of the infection and fight it. *H. pylori*, however, attaches itself to these sugar cells and in so doing is able to move more deeply in the stomach wall. Because the white blood cells can't fight the *H. pylori* infection, the infection grows even stronger, the stomach produces more sugar molecules in a louder cry for help, and the infection grows stronger still. Over time, a buildup of white blood cells occurs because the stomach keeps asking for them, but the cells are unable to penetrate the mucosal layer. In this cycle of continuously reinforced infection, the stomach lining becomes inflamed. Some researchers believe that this inflammation of the stomach—not *H. pylori*—is responsible for ulcers.

H. PYLORI AND DUODENAL ULCERS

H. pylori is responsible for 70 to 80 percent of stomach ulcers (with NSAIDs taking the rest of the blame), but the bacterium is responsible for 90 to 95 percent of duodenal ulcers. These ulcers occur in the duodenum, the first part of the small intestine. Stomach acid is neutralized in the duodenum. The bile duct and pancreatic duct open into the duodenum and deliver bile from the liver and enzymes from the pancreas. These substances aid in digestion. The duodenum's job is to process food into smaller pieces so that it can pass through the wall of the small intestine, be absorbed in the bloodstream, and nourish the body.

Ninety-five percent of duodenal ulcers occur in the duodenal bulb, or cap, the first portion of the duodenum. Like the epithelial cells in the stomach, epithelial cells in the duodenum produce mucus to protect against damage by gastric acid and pepsinogen. Normally, H. pylori bacteria do not colonize the duodenum's mucus layer. However, H. pylori infections in the stomach can produce unusually high amounts of acid, and this causes more acid to spill into the duodenum. To protect against this acid influx, the epithelial cells in the duodenum undergo a transformation, or metaplasia. These duodenum cells are replaced by the kind of epithelial cells found in the stomach. Because H. pylori can infect the mucus produced by these cells, the duodenum is subject to the same H. pylori problems as the stomach. The duodenum can be infected by H. pylori, resulting in duodenitis or a duodenal ulcer.

WHY ARE MOST PEOPLE SPARED?

One of the biggest enigmas surrounding H. pylori is why only one in six people infected with the bacteria gets a peptic disease or ulcer. By far, the majority of infected people show no ill effects whatsoever. Why is that?

One reason has to do with H. pylori bacterial strains. Some strains are more virulent than others. Microarray analysis, a kind of genetic fingerprinting, now allows scientists to examine the different gene sequences in a microorganism. Using microarray analysis, scientists have determined that three-fourths of the genes in *H. pylori* bacterium strains are identical, but a quarter of the gene sequences are specific to each strain. This leaves a lot of room for diversity among *H. pylori* strains.

One gene, called *cagA* (Cytotoxin-associated gene), has been identified in connection with the virulent *H. pylori* strains that cause gastritis. Patients infected with *H. pylori* strains that include the *cagA* gene are more likely to suffer from chronic inflammation of the stomach, peptic ulcer disease, and duodenal ulcers. In Asia, where infection rates are high, 95 percent of *H. pylori* strains contain *cagA*. At present, microbiologists are examining the genes in the different *H. pylori* strains, and the coming years will probably reveal much about the virulence of the different strains and determine which ones are responsible for peptic ulcers.

Another reason that some people are spared is based upon the theory that the *H. pylori* bacterium doesn't cause ulcers. *H. pylori* is an opportunistic bacterium that attacks tissue that has already been inflamed or damaged; it isn't the disease agent. Of course, diet, smoking, and environmental factors also play a role in whether an *H. pylori* infection leads to full-blown gastritis or an ulcer. And older people are more susceptible to ulcers than others, especially if they have been harboring the *H. pylori* bacteria since childhood or they are taking NSAIDs.

Perhaps the physicians of fifty years ago who believed that stress causes ulcers were not entirely wrong. Whether *H. pylori* bacteria cause an ulcer has much to do with a person's immune system. A vibrant immune system confronts and defeats literally billions of germs each day, *H. pylori* included. Stress does play a role in whether you get an ulcer because chronic stress weakens the immune system, which in turn can make you more susceptible to an infection by *H. pylori* or another bacterium.

DIAGNOSING *H. PYLORI* INFECTIONS

Because the majority of people who are infected with *H. pylori* do not develop an ulcer disease, most doctors do not test for *H. pylori* infections in every patient with symptoms of an ulcer. Usually, tests are given initially only to people over the age of 50 who have a history of peptic ulcer disease, patients with a family member who has had an ulcer or stomach cancer, and those who have had recent bouts of dyspepsia.

The three categories of tests for the presence of the bacterium include: Procedures such as an endoscopy for examining the upper gastrointestinal (GI) tract and obtaining tissue biopsies; biopsy tests for detecting the presence of *H. pylori* in tissue; and noninvasive tests. All of these diagnostic tests are explained in detail in Chapter 5. Diagnostic tests and procedures specific to *H. pylori* infections are briefly described here.

Meanwhile, to have a successful *H. pylori* diagnostic test and avoid a false-negative test result, patients (except for those taking blood tests and undergoing endoscopies) must observe these rules:

- No eating for six hours before the test.

- No taking antacid tablets for two weeks before the test.

- No taking proton pump inhibitors for two weeks before the test.

- No taking H_2 blockers for two weeks before the test.

- No taking antibiotics for one month before the test.

- No taking bismuth (Pepto Bismol) for one month before the test.

Be sure to consult your physician before you take a diagnostic test to make sure that you prepare yourself correctly.

Endoscopy

In an endoscopy, also known as a gastroscopy, the patient is lightly sedated and an endoscope, a fiber-optic tube with a tiny camera on the end, is eased into the patient's throat to the stomach and duodenum. Doctors can view and take pictures of the patient's esophagus, stomach, and duodenum through an endoscope. By means of small forceps on the instrument, doctors can remove tissue samples, which can then be examined for the presence of *H. pylori* bacteria.

An endoscopy offers the most thorough diagnosis of *H. pylori* infection, but the procedure must be performed in a clinic or hospital, and at $1,000 plus the cost of subsequent testing, it is expensive. An endoscopy takes ten to fifteen minutes. Some patients find the fiber-optic tube—about the width of a little finger—very uncomfortable.

Biopsy Tests

After a tissue sample has been obtained by endoscopy, doctors can conduct the following tests to see if the tissue is infected by *H. pylori:*

- **Rapid urease test (RUT).** A tissue sample is placed in agar gel containing urea and a pH-sensitive indicator. If the tissue contains *H. pylori* bacteria, the bacteria's urease enzymes react to the urea and change the color of the gel. Test results can be obtained in one day.

- ***H. pylori* culture.** The tissue is placed in an agar plate, and, if bacteria are present, they are cultured and studied. Doctors use this time-consuming and expensive testing method when antibiotic therapy fails and they want to investigate an *H. pylori* strain for sensitivity to antibiotics.

- **Histologic assessment.** The tissue sample is stained with different dyes for identification purposes and then examined under a microscope for *H. pylori* infection.

- **Polymerase chain reaction (PCR) assay.** Samples are copied by means of PCR, a technique for examining DNA, and then analyzed for *H. pylori* genes.

The test your doctor chooses for you will depend on cost, his or her assessment of the degree to which you are infected by *H. pylori,* and other factors.

Noninvasive Tests

The following noninvasive tests are not as accurate as the others, but they submit patients to less discomfort and provide results much earlier:

- **Urea breath.** Detects urease in the patient's lungs. Urease is an enzyme produced by *H. pylori*. If urease is detected, *H. pylori* are present in the patient's GI tract.

- **Serological (antibody).** Detects *H. pylori* antibodies in the patient's blood. Patients with these antibodies may be infected. Because antibodies remain in the blood after the bacteria are eradicated, a positive test result doesn't necessarily mean that the patient is infected.

- **Finger-prick blood test.** Detects anti-*H. pylori* antibodies in whole blood obtained by pricking the skin.

- **Stool antigen immunoassay.** Detects *H. pylori* antigens in stool. An antigen is any substance that provokes the immune system to respond.

- **Saliva.** Detects *H. pylori* in saliva samples.

These tests do not require taking a tissue sample by endoscopy. They are often given to patients who cannot bear having an endoscopy tube in their throat and stomach.

THE HERETICAL VIEW:
H. PYLORI IS GOOD FOR YOUR ESOPHAGUS

So far, I have discussed the numerous disadvantages of being infected with *H. pylori* bacteria. It causes gastritis. The bacterium can cause stomach ulcers and ulcers of the duodenum. It may cause stomach cancer. In spite of all that, some scientists have speculated that there may be health benefits to being infected with *H. pylori*. They base this idea on the fact that the bacteria have infected the majority of humankind for many millennia. That being so, wouldn't the body have rid itself of *H. pylori* by now if the bacteria didn't offer some health advantages? As stomach ulcer rates and stomach cancer rates decline in the United States, rates of esophageal diseases, cancer of the esophagus, and GERD (gastroesophageal reflux disease) are rising, especially among white men. The esophagus is the swallowing tube that connects your mouth to your stomach. Could the eradication of *H. pylori* bacteria have something to do with the increase in esophageal diseases, GERD, and esophageal cancer?

In a study conducted in Essen, Germany, doctors tracked patients who had been treated for *H. pylori* infection to see whether they were more likely to get reflux esophagitis (an inflammation of the esophagus that can cause difficulty swallowing), heartburn, and sometimes bleeding. Reflux esophagitis results from stomach acid backing up into the esophagus and causing irritation. The German doctors discovered that patients who had been rid of *H. pylori* were twice as likely as patients who harbor the bacteria to have reflux esophagitis.

In a similar study conducted at the National Cancer Institute in Bethesda, Maryland, scientists determined that people infected with *cagA* (Cytotoxin-associated gene) strains of *H. pylori* were less likely to get cancer of the esophagus. As I explained earlier in this chapter, *cagA* is a gene found in particularly virulent strains of *H. pylori*. Finally, in a 2003 study that was conducted at the Oregon Health and Science University in Portland, Oregon, scientists determined that *cagA* strains of *H. pylori* encourage cancerous cells in the esophagus to self-destruct by apoptosis (disintegration), but leave healthy esophageal cells alone.

The number of esophageal cancers is increasing in the United States at the rate of 8 to 9 percent annually. Incidences of esophageal cancer are increasing faster than any other cancer. Some researchers believe that the aggressive treatment of *H. pylori* infections with antibiotics is causing this inflation of esophageal cancer rates. With *H. pylori* chased from the scene, cancerous cells in the esophagus get the chance to grow and multiply.

If it is, in fact, true that harboring *H. pylori* is healthy for the esophagus, doctors will face a dilemma when treating patients with *H. pylori* infections. They will have to carefully weigh the benefits against the costs of eradicating *H. pylori*. Patients who today are given antibiotics to treat nonulcerative dyspepsia, for example, may not be treated with antibiotics in the future. Doctors may decide that the slight improvement these patients may experince from antibiotic treatment is not worth the risk of getting cancer of the esophagus.

In the future, *H. pylori* may be called a "colonizer," not an infectious agent, considering that the bacterium may offer health bene-fits to the esophagus. At any rate, whether the bacterium turns out to be a colonizer or an infectious agent, the *H. pylori* mystery is a fascinating one.

CONCLUSION

The 1983 discovery of *H. pylori* by Australian scientists Barry Mar-shall and Robin Warren caused doctors everywhere to rethink their ideas about peptic ulcer disease. It took ten years, but the medical community finally came around to the Australian scientists' way of thinking, and now the eradication of *H. pylori* bacteria with antibiotics is the first line of treatment for peptic ulcer disease.

While eradicating *H. pylori* with antibiotics has cured many patients of their ulcers, it has brought along a new set of problems for doctors to consider. The widespread use of antibiotics encour-ages new *H. pylori* strains to evolve—and some of these strains are already proving resistant to antibiotics. In addition, antibiotic treat-ment does not guarantee that a patient will remain uninfected, since patients may pick up *H. pylori* bacteria again, especially if they live in unsanitary conditions.

The *H. pylori* bacterium is the chief cause of peptic ulcer disease worldwide and will remain so in the developing world, where san-itary conditions permit the bacteria to spread. The industrialized world is another story. In the United States and Europe, where good sanitary conditions prevail, another culprit is slowly creep-ing up as the primary cause of peptic ulcer disease. That culprit is NSAIDs, or non-steroidal anti-inflammatory drugs, which will likely cause increasing amounts of peptic ulcer disease in the industrialized world in the years to come. The next chapter focus-es on NSAIDs and looks at how these drugs cause ulcers.

3

NSAIDs and Ulcers

pproximately 25 percent of chronic users of NSAIDs (pronounced EN-seds) develop a peptic ulcer. After the bacterium *Helicobacter pylori* (*H. pylori*), NSAIDs—non-steroidal anti-inflammatory drugs—are the leading cause of peptic ulcer disease. In the United States, gastrointestinal complications caused by NSAIDs are responsible for 16,500 deaths annually and more than 100,000 hospitalizations. In this chapter, I will be taking a closer look at NSAIDS, explaining what they are and how they work. I'll present their harmful side effects, and show how they can damage the gastrointestinal tract. I'll also detail the symptoms of NSAID-induced ulcers, as well as the risk factors for developing this condition.

As the previous chapter explained, the number of people infected with the *H. pylori* bacterium decreases with each successive generation, at least in the United States and the rest of the industrialized world. If this trend continues, fewer people will be infected with *H. pylori* in the United States, and, in a generation or two, NSAIDs will become the primary cause of peptic ulcer disease. For that reason, understanding why NSAIDs cause ulcers and learning how to treat NSAID-induced ulcers has taken on a new urgency.

THE NSAIDS IN YOUR MEDICINE CABINET

Non-steroidal anti-inflammatory drugs are used as pain relievers;

to treat inflammatory conditions such as arthritis, bursitis, and tendonitis; to reduce fevers; and to thin the blood to protect against heart attacks and strokes. Many NSAIDs are sold over-the-counter. In the United States alone, more than 30 billion over-the-counter NSAID tablets are purchased annually. Pharmacists fill 70 million NSAID prescriptions each year. Whether you know it or not, you almost certainly have at least one NSAID in your medicine cabinet. Ibuprofen (Advil, Motrin), for example, is a nonsteroidal anti-inflammatory drug. The best-known NSAID is aspirin. This drug has been sold over-the-counter in the United States since 1915. According to Bayer, Americans take 80 million aspirin pills a day. Sales of NSAIDs amount to about $2 billion per year.

Table 3.1 on the next page lists popular NSAIDs by their generic names and brand names. In the table, entries that are marked with an asterisk (*) are COX-2 inhibitor NSAIDs, and they are explained later in the chapter. By the way, acetaminophen (Tylenol, Exdol, Panadol, Paracetamol) is not an NSAID. It is effective against pain and fever, but not against inflammation or pain caused by inflammation, and its mode of action is different from that of an NSAID.

A "SILENT EPIDEMIC"

Taking the occasional NSAID does no harm, but taking the drugs habitually puts you at risk for getting a peptic ulcer. You may also be at risk for other conditions such as kidney problems, fluid retention, miscarriage, and excessive bleeding. The June 1999 issue of the *New England Journal of Medicine* called deaths caused by NSAIDs a "silent epidemic." The journal called attention to the fact that as many people die from ulcers caused by NSAIDs as from myeloma, asthma, cervical cancer, or Hodgkin's disease. "If deaths from gastrointestinal toxic effects from NSAIDs were tabulated separately in the National Vital Statistics reports," the *Journal* pointed out, "these effects would constitute the fifteenth most common cause of death in the United States."

Consider the following statistics (found on page 48) regarding NSAID-caused death and illness:

TABLE 3.1. NON-STEROIDAL ANTI-INFLAMMATORY DRUGS (NSAIDS)	
GENERIC NAME	BRAND NAME
acetylsalicylic acid (ASA)	Anacin, aspirin
celecoxib*	Celebrex
diclofenac	Apo-Diclo, Novo-Difenac, Voltaren
diflunisal	Dolobid
etodolac	Lodine, Ultradol
fenoprofen	Nalfon
fluribuprofen	Ansaid, Froben
ibuprofen	Advil, Motrin, Nuprin
indomethacin	Apo-Indomethacin, Indocid, Novo-Methacin
ketoprofen	Apo-Keto-E, Novo-Profen, Orudis, Oruvail, Rhodis
ketorolac	Toradol
meloxicam	Mobicox
nabumetone	Relafen
naproxen	Aleve, Anaprox, Apo-Naproxen, Naprosyn, Naxen, Novo-Naprox
oxaprozin	Daypro
piroxicam	Apo-Piroxicam, Feldene, Novo-Pirocam
rofecoxib*	Vioxx
salsalate	Disalcid
sulindac	Aclin, Apo-Sulin, Clinoril, Novo-Sudac
tenoxicam	Mobiflex
tiaprofenic acid	AlbertTiafen, Surgam
tolmetin	Tolectin
valdecoxib*	Bextra

* COX-2 inhibitor NSAID

- By conservative estimates, over 100,000 Americans are hospitalized each year for NSAID-related gastrointestinal complications.

- The cost of treating the side effects from NSAIDs is approximately $20 billion annually.

- People who use NSAIDs are five to twenty times more likely than others to get peptic ulcer disease. In people who are infected with the *H. pylori* bacterium, the risk is five to seven times higher.

- Some studies show that 25 percent of arthritis patients who habitually use NSAIDs develop an ulcer.

NSAIDs can be purchased over-the-counter. They are inexpensive and easy to take orally. They work fast. For all these reasons, it is easy to abuse NSAIDs. However, the public is not cognizant of how dangerous taking NSAIDs for long periods of time can be, especially for the elderly. In a 1998 survey of 5,000 people conducted by the American Gastroenterological Association (AGA) to gauge the public's understanding of NSAIDs, the AGA discovered that three-quarters of Americans don't realize that NSAIDs can be harmful. This remarkable finding illustrates how NSAIDs are so well marketed. The public understands the pills' benefits, but, clearly is ignorant of the drugs' sometimes-hazardous side effects.

If NSAIDs are so bad for you, why do doctors continue to prescribe them and patients continue to take them? The answer is that the drugs offer enormous benefits, especially to elderly people who suffer from osteoarthritis. NSAIDs are useful against arthritis, fevers, migraines, post-operative pain, and even Alzheimer's disease and colon polyps. In low doses, aspirin can help prevent heart attacks and strokes. NSAIDs would probably be considered wonder drugs if not for the fact that they can cause ulcers and other harmful conditions. Whenever doctors consider prescribing an NSAID, they must carefully weight the benefits of the drug against its side effects. To minimize the risks, doctors usually prescribe the lowest effective dose for the shortest possible duration—but this may not always be the case.

Aspirin: The World's First Wonder Drug

It is often said of aspirin that if the drug were invented today, the Federal Drug Administration (FDA) would ban it. Aspirin couldn't withstand the rigorous testing that the FDA requires of modern drugs. It would cause the death of too many in vitro test-tube cells. It would ulcerate and kill too many laboratory rats. Aspirin has too many dangerous side effects and its action isn't entirely understood. Fortunately for headache sufferers, however, aspirin was "grandfathered" into the modern pharmacopeia. It has been a staple on drugstore shelves for nearly a century.

Aspirin's origins can be traced to the bark of the beautiful white willow tree. Ground down into a powder form, willow tree bark was used as a medicine for pain and fever. This effective folk remedy was used by the Chickasaw Indians of North America, the ancient Chinese, and numerous cultures in between. The man for whom the Hippocratic Oath is named wasn't afraid to confer with traditional healers and find out how they treated their patients. In the fifth century B.C.E., Hippocrates wrote of a bitter powder extract from willow bark that traditional healers used to relieve labor and inflammatory pain.

The discovery of aspirin is usually credited to the Reverend Edmund Stone of Chipping Norton in Oxfordshire, England. In 1763, Reverend Stone wrote to the president of the Royal Society in London, describing how he had successfully treated "over 50 patients suffering from various agues" (fevers) by means of powdered bark from the white willow tree. It took the work of several European chemists to turn the Reverend Stone's willow bark into aspirin. In 1828, Johann Buchner, a professor at the University of Munich, isolated the yellow crystals in willow bark that are responsible for giving pain relief. He called these crystals salicin, from salix, the Latin word for "willow." In 1838, Raffaele Piria, an Italian chemist working at the Sorbonne, succeeded in turning salicin into salicylic acid. Salicylic acid was used in high doses to treat arthritis and other inflammatory ailments, influenza, and fever. Unfortunately, but predictably, the treatment often proved worse than the cure. Patients who managed to swallow the bitter salicylic acid without gagging often developed stomach ulcers.

The problem for chemists was how to buffer salicylic acid so it could be absorbed without causing too much harm to the stomach. In 1853, a French chemist named Charles Frederic Gerhardt succeeded in buffering aspirin. Gerhardt created acetylsalicylic acid (ASA), the substance we know today as "aspirin." By buffering salicylic acid with sodium and acetyl chloride, he was able to neutralize salicylic acid's harmful effects. Gerhardt shelved his discovery, thinking it wasn't worth pursuing, and forty-four years later the magic formula was rediscovered by the brilliant German chemist Felix Hoffmann. Hoffman synthesized the first aspirin for his ailing rheumatic father. The drug worked wonders and was easily tolerated.

The chemist had trouble convincing his employers at Friedrich Bayer & Co. to develop the new drug. His employers were more enthusiastic for another Hoffmann creation—the drug heroin. Hoffmann gave aspirin to patients in Berlin hospitals, and on the strength of those early trials, Bayer took out the first patent for aspirin in 1899. Bayer chose the name as follows: the "a" comes from acetyl chloride; the "spir" comes from spiraea ulmaria, the plant from which the salicylic acid used in production comes (many plants make salicylic acid, not just the willow); and "in" was a common ending for medicine names a hundred years ago.

Bayer's prescription aspirin powder proved successful from the start. By 1915, aspirin was being sold over-the-counter in tablets in the United States. Bayer held the trademark on aspirin until the conclusion of World War I, when the German company relinquished its trademark to pay war reparations as part of the Treaty of Versailles. Immediately, other drug companies began manufacturing untrademarked aspirin, one of the most successful medicines of all time.

HOW NSAIDS WORK

Until fairly recently, taking NSAIDs was an act of faith. People took the drugs without understanding how or why they relieved pain and swelling. The 1982 Nobel Prize in Medicine was awarded to three scientists—John Vane, Sune Bergstrom, and Bengt Samuelsson—who are credited for understanding how aspirin works. They discovered aspirin's ability to stop the production of prostaglandins.

Stopping Prostaglandins

NSAIDs, including aspirin, work by affecting substances in the body called *prostaglandins*. These potent hormone-like substances play many important roles. They serve as messenger molecules to tell the brain when a part of the body has been injured. They are involved in creating the mucus that protects the lining of the stomach and duodenum. They help to constrict the uterus during labor. They are involved in the inflammatory process. They participate in the aggregation of platelets that causes blood clotting. They may also play a role in the formation of tumors. Prostaglandins owe their name to the prostate gland. In the 1930s, researchers under the direction of young Dr. Ulf von Euler discovered prostaglandins in semen, so they assumed that the molecules were produced in the prostate gland. However, prostaglandins are produced in the cell membranes of nearly every body tissue.

When you receive a bodily injury or get an infection, the injured cells produce high concentrations of prostaglandins. In injuries and infections, prostaglandins perform two important tasks. First, along with other chemicals, they transmit messages to your brain telling it when a part of your body needs care and healing. The message goes something like this: "It hurts." You feel pain, and you know to take care of the cut on your finger, your headache, or whatever ails you. Second, prostaglandins cause blood vessels to dilate at the site of the injury or infection. This permits more blood to flow through and nurse the wounded tissue. More white blood cells and other healing agents can come to the site of the injury through the bloodstream. The downside, however, is that swelling occurs to accommodate this excess blood, and, as anyone who has ever sprained an ankle or wrist knows, swelling hurts.

People take aspirin, ibuprofen, and other NSAIDs to lessen pain and decrease the swelling of body tissue. The drug dissolves in the stomach, passes through the walls of the small intestine, and enters the bloodstream. From there, it finds where prostaglandins are being produced in high concentrations, and then it stops their production. The result is a reduction in pain and swelling. The headache goes away. The cut on the finger doesn't hurt as badly. The sprained ankle doesn't throb as painfully as it used to. The discomfort of fever is lessened. NSAIDs don't heal injuries or infections, but they stop prostaglandin production to relieve the pain and swelling that accompanies injuries and infections.

Seems perfect, right? Not quite. The trouble with taking an NSAID is that the drug affects prostaglandins throughout the body, not just those at the site of a wound or infection. For the purposes of this book, what matters most is that NSAIDs also block the prostaglandins in the stomach that stimulate mucus production. This is why NSAIDs irritate the stomach and cause ulcers. With fewer prostaglandins to simulate the production of mucus, the stomach's mucosal protection is weakened, and the stomach is more susceptible to ulcers and to being scalded by acid. Most of the harmful side effects of NSAIDs occur because prostaglandins figure in so many body functions and NSAIDs affect prostaglandins in nearly every part of the body.

Interfering with the COX Enzymes

The mechanism by which NSAIDs stop the production of prostaglandins is important to understand because it bears on the development of a new class of NSAIDs called COX-2 inhibitors.

NSAIDs achieve their effects by interfering with an enzyme called cyclooxygenase, or COX for short. Normally, COX enzymes convert arachidonic acid— an essential fatty acid that is absorbed with food and found mainly in red meat, egg yolks, and organ meats—into prostaglandins. NSAIDs, however, prevent COX enzymes from converting arachidonic acid into prostaglandins. NSAIDs do this by attaching themselves to the receptors on arachidonic acid so that COX enzymes can't access them. In effect, NSAIDs come between COX enzymes and arachidonic acid so that the production of prostaglandins is halted.

Scientists have identified three types of COX enzymes. The COX-1 enzyme is involved in creating the maintenance prostaglandins that regulate pain, blood clotting, blood flow to the kidneys, and mucus production in the stomach. COX-1 is present in most body tissue cells. Levels of COX-1 remain stable. To use a biochemical term, the enzyme is *constitutive*, which means that its concentration levels in body tissue do not change.

The COX-2 enzyme is involved in creating prostaglandins that manage the inflammatory process and the pain associated with inflammation. Normally, COX-2 is not present in cells, but COX-2 levels increase dramatically as part of the immune system's response to injuries and infections. To use the biochemical term, COX-2 enzymes are *inducible*. When you get a wound or infection, COX-2 concentration levels increase at the site of the injury. It appears that macrophages, the large white blood cells that attack bacteria and other pathogens, stimulate the production of COX-2 enzymes.

The COX-3 enzyme appears to create prostaglandins in the brain and spinal cord that regulate pain and fever. COX-3 was discovered quite recently as part of an investigation into the drug acetaminophen (Tylenol, Exdol, Panadol, Paracetamol). This drug—which is not an NSAID—is a good painkiller. Unlike an NSAID, it doesn't affect the protective lining of the stomach. Acetaminophen has little effect on COX-1 and COX-2 enzymes. Researchers speculate that acetaminophen relieves pain and fever by targeting COX-3. As of this publication, however, research into the COX-3 enzyme is still in the infancy stage.

After scientists discovered the different kinds of COX enzymes, drug companies set to work trying to invent NSAIDs that would affect the COX-2 enzymes associated with pain, but not the COX-1 enzymes associated with mucus production in the stomach. The idea was to relieve pain and joint inflammation without harming the stomach or causing ulcers. This new class of NSAIDs is called COX-2 inhibitors.

COX-2 INHIBITOR NSAIDS

In 1999, drug manufacturers introduced a class of NSAIDs called COX-2 inhibitors (sometimes called COX-2 selective inhibitors). The drugs were bestsellers from the start. Arthritis sufferers were eager to take medications that eased joint pain without causing gastrointestinal pain, bleeding, and the other common side effects associated with NSAIDs. In the year after COX-2 inhibitors were introduced, doctors wrote over 100 million prescriptions for celecoxib (Celebrex) and rofecoxib (Vioxx). Celebrex is now one of the top-selling drugs, with sales of more than $4 billion since its debut in 1999. Vioxx, the other best-selling COX-2 inhibitor, had sales amounting to $2.5 billion in 2001.

The idea behind COX-2 inhibitors is to offer people with rheumatoid arthritis the benefits of NSAIDs without the harmful side effects. As I explained, NSAIDs work by halting the production of prostaglandins, and to do that, they interrupt the activity of COX-1 and COX-2 enzymes. Most of the harmful side effects of NSAIDs result from the interruption of COX-1 enzymes. Among other things, COX-1 enzymes help produce the mucus in the stomach lining that protects the stomach against ulcers. COX-2 inhibitors only affect—or inhibit—the COX-2 enzymes that bring about pain and inflammation; they leave the COX-1 enzymes involved in stomach mucus production alone.

In theory, this class of drug inhibits only COX-2 enzymes, but in practice, the jury is still deliberating. COX-2 inhibitors may also erode the stomach's mucus protection, although the drugs are not as harmful to the gastrointestinal tract as other NSAIDs. Like other NSAIDs, the drugs may damage the kidneys. Some physicians believe that COX-2 inhibitors increase the risk of heart attacks and strokes. Others have called into question the drugs' benefits given how expensive they are compared to other NSAIDs. COX-2 inhibitors cost roughly $2.75 per tablet—significantly more than naproxen, for example, which costs $.18 per tablet.

Much to the displeasure of Pharmacia and Merck (the makers of Celebrex and Vioxx), the Federal Drug Administration (FDA) requires COX-2 inhibitor drugs to carry the same gastrointestinal risk warning as other NSAIDs. In February 2000, on the strength of new studies they had commissioned, Pharmacia and Merck asked the Arthritis Advisory Committee to the FDA to review whether these warnings were necessary. The Committee concluded that the studies did not show that COX-2 inhibitors have a "clinically meaningful" safety advantage over standard NSAIDs, nor did they show an overall reduction in gastrointestinal complications. The gastrointestinal health warnings remain on the labels of COX-2 inhibitors.

NSAIDs decrease blood flow to the kidneys, and for that reason, they have been linked to kidney failure, especially in elderly patients and patients with pre-existing kidney damage. COX-2 inhibitors, it appears, are no different from other NSAIDs in their effect on the kidneys. In a study published in the July 4, 2000 *Annals of Internal Medicine,* researchers had seventy-five patients aged 60 to 80 years with normally functioning kidneys take the COX-2 inhibitor rofecoxib (Vioxx), the NSAID indomethacin (Apo-Indomethacin, Indocid, Novo-Methacin), or a placebo. Subjects in all three groups were placed on a low-sodium diet because salt intake can affect test results in renal studies. To gauge the subjects' kidney health, researchers examined sodium levels and potassium levels in the subjects' urine and blood. In groups taking the COX-2 inhibitor and the NSAID, the subjects' ability to filter waste products declined to the same degree. The authors of the study concluded, "the renal effects observed . . . are likely to be reproduced throughout this class of medications." In other words, COX-2 inhibitors are as likely as standard NSAIDs to cause kidney problems.

Another troubling aspect of COX-2 inhibitors is their potential to increase the risk of heart attacks and strokes. In 2001, cardiologists at the Cleveland Clinic analyzed clinical trials of COX-2 inhibitors to determine if these drugs have any effect on cardiovascular health. In a trial involving 8,059 people with rheumatoid arthritis who were given the COX-2 inhibitor rofecoxib (Vioxx) or the NSAID diclofenac, patients taking the COX-2 inhibitor were twice as likely to have a heart attack, stroke, or other cardiovascular event. This trial was supposed to exclude people who had a history of heart disease, but it so happened that 321 subjects with heart disease were included in the study by mistake. Among these people, those who took the COX-2 inhibitor were four times more likely to have a cardiovascular event. This trial was significant because, during the trial, subjects weren't permitted to take aspirin, a drug known to protect against heart attacks.

The Cleveland Clinic also looked at a trial involving roughly 8,000 patients who took celecoxib (Celebrex) or an NSAID. Patients were allowed to take aspirin during this trial. The trial revealed no difference in cardiovascular events between the group taking COX-2 inhibitors and the group taking standard NSAIDs, but this may have been attributable to the patients' taking aspirin, according to the Cleveland Clinic.

Neither trial that the Cleveland Clinic analyzed was initially designed to investigate cardiovascular events (the trials were designed to compare the effect of COX-2 inhibitors and NSAIDs on the gastrointestinal tract). Moreover, although the drugs double the risk of getting a heart attack, the risk remains quite low.

Still, these trials raise concerns because they point to something in COX-2 inhibitors that can cause heart disease. As early as 1999, the National Academy of Science warned that COX-2 inhibitors increase the risk of strokes, heart attacks, and blood-clotting disorders. One theory is that COX-2 inhibitors suppress the production of prostacyclin, a prostaglandin in the walls of blood vessels that acts to dilate the vessels and inhibit blood clots. The FDA is so concerned that COX-2 inhibitors increase the risk of heart attacks that the agency's Health and Human Services Department cited Merck (the maker of Vioxx) in a September 21, 2001 warning letter. Merck, the agency wrote, has "engaged in a promotional campaign for Vioxx that minimizes the potentially serious cardiovascular findings that were observed . . . and thus, misrepresents the safety profile for Vioxx."

Finally, the high cost of COX-2 inhibitors relative to other NSAIDs has caused some to question whether the drugs are cost-effective. In some studies, the absolute risk reduction of taking COX-2 inhibitors is only 1 or 2 percent compared to other NSAIDs. If the risk reduction is this low, is spending an extra $500 to $700 a year for COX-2 inhibitors worthwhile? To measure the cost-effectiveness of COX-2 inhibitors, researchers at UCLA and the VA Greater Los Angeles Healthcare System devised a QALY (quality-adjusted life-year) measurement scale for a hypothetical 60-year-old patient with mild to severe arthritic pain. Without going into the details, the study found that COX-2 inhibitors cost $275,809 more than naproxen to produce each additional QALY. For patients with heart disease, COX-2 inhibitors cost $395,324 more. The authors concluded: "The risk reduction seen with coxibs (COX-2 inhibitors) does not offset their increased costs compared with nonselective NSAIDs in the management of average-risk patients with chronic arthritis. However, coxibs may provide an acceptable incremental cost-effectiveness ratio in the subgroup of patients with a history of bleeding ulcers."

It has been suggested that COX-2 inhibitors were placed on the market before sufficient studies were done on their effectiveness, and that the drugs were pushed forward too quickly by pharmaceutical companies. Larry Sasich, a pharmacist for the Public Citizen Health Research Group, put it this way: "The question prescribers have to ask is how did Celebrex reach $1 billion in sales at a time when there wasn't a single controlled trial published that looked at the effectiveness in treating arthritis and pain compared to similar drugs. What sources of information do prescribers use to choose drugs? In the case of Celebrex, because there was no science, the decision had to be based on promotional materials."

ASSESSING THE RISK OF DIFFERENT NSAIDS

Needless to say, arthritis sufferers are better off taking the NSAIDs that cause the least harm to their gastrointestinal tracts. Even among standard NSAIDs, there are some that behave more like COX-2 inhibitors, in that they interfere more with the COX-2 enzymes that have to do with inflammatory pain and less with the COX-1 enzymes that create mucosal protection in the stomach. Scientists use the terms "COX-1 selective" and "COX-2 selective" to describe the effect of NSAIDs on respective COX-1 and COX-2 enzymes. The ideal NSAID would be entirely COX-2 selective because it would interfere only with the COX-2 enzymes involved in inflammatory pain; it would disregard the COX-1 enzymes that help protect the stomach against ulcers. However, no such NSAID exists. On the COX-1 selective, COX-2 selective scale, all NSAIDs fall somewhere between the two extremes.

Many studies have been done to try to find out where NSAIDs are on the scale and which NSAIDs cause the most gastrointestinal distress. Unfortunately, the studies sometimes contradict one another. In addition, methods for measuring if an NSAID is COX-1 selective or COX-2 selective is imprecise. However, a general reading of various studies reveals the following:

- The standard NSAIDs that are most harmful to the stomach are indomethacin, sulindac, piroxicam, and aspirin.

- The COX-2 inhibitor NSAIDs that are least harmful to the stomach are ibuprofen, nabumetone, ketorolac, and etodolac.

If your doctor wants to prescribe an NSAID, be sure to ask what the risks of the particular NSAID are to your gastrointestinal health.

HOW NSAIDS CAUSE PEPTIC ULCERS

NSAIDs weaken the stomach in two different ways. When they arrive in the stomach, they cause topical damage to the stomach's interior lining. Most of the damage done by NSAIDs, however, occurs systemically after the drug enters the bloodstream. Traveling in the bloodstream, NSAIDs locate where prostaglandins are being produced and halt the production of those prostaglandins. Prostaglandins in the stomach figure in the creation of mucus for the stomach's protection, but NSAIDs hinder the protective mucus from forming. The result can be an ulcer.

Topical Damage

In medical terminology, "topical" pertains to a particular surface area. To begin with, NSAIDs cause topical damage to the interior surface of the stomach. These drugs are weak organic acids. They are soluble (dissolvable) in lipids (fat). Cell membranes in the surface epithelial cells of the stomach lining contain lipids, whose job is to protect against gastric acid. Because NSAIDs can dissolve into these lipids, they can pass through the cell walls and become trapped inside the lipid membranes of the stomach's epithelial cells. As NSAID compounds become concentrated in these cells, a toxic effect ensues. The cells become more permeable. They swell and die in greater numbers.

Within an hour of ingesting a single dose of aspirin, tiny superficial lesions and hemorrhages—most of which occur in the fundus, the convex upper portion of the stomach—appear on the stomach lining. After repeated doses of aspirin, gastric erosions also begin appearing in the antrum, the area of the stomach immediately before the small intestine. This sounds a lot worse than it really is. Fortunately, the tiny lesions disappear after a while in a rather mysterious process known as gastric adaptation. The gastric erosions usually subside when a person continues to take aspirin for several days, and, in about four weeks, the erosions usually disappear.

Studies of the initial, topical damage done by NSAIDs to the epithelial cells—that is, those cells forming the stomach lining—have not shown conclusively whether this initial damage increases a patient's chances of getting a stomach ulcer. The majority of physicians believe that NSAID-caused topical damage is not clinically meaningful. In other words, topical damage in the stomach is not a significant or necessary step in the development of a stomach ulcer. The alternate view, however, is that topical injuries caused by NSAIDs deplete prostaglandins and expose the stomach to greater harm from gastric acid. For those reasons, some physicians believe that NSAID-caused topical injury is an important component of stomach ulcers.

Systemic Damage

In medical terminology, "systemic" refers to something that reaches cells throughout the body. Most physicians agree that NSAIDs damage the body systemically by interfering with prostaglandin production. Earlier in this chapter, I explained how hormone-like substances called prostaglandins help create the gel-like mucus layer that protects the stomach and duodenum against gastric acid (see "Stopping Prostaglandins" beginning on page 50). NSAIDs cause ulcers by interfering with prostaglandin production, and impairing the stomach's mucosal defense. The evidence is very convincing:

- Patients given synthetic prostaglandins along with NSAIDs do not develop ulcers at the same rate as other patients who take NSAIDs. In a double-blind, placebo-controlled study conducted in 1988 at the Veterans Administration Medical Center in Houston, Texas, 420 patients taking NSAIDs with osteoarthritis were given a placebo or two hundred micrograms of the synthetic prostaglandin misoprostol (Cytotec) four times daily. By 1.4 percent to 21.7 percent, gastric ulcers occurred less frequently in the misoprostol group than in the placebo group.

- In experiments, animals were given antibodies, which halted prostaglandin production. The absence of prostaglandins caused stomach ulcers.

- Patients who take COX-2 inhibitors—NSAIDs designed to leave prostaglandins in the stomach and duodenum alone—do not acquire ulcers at the same rate as patients taking standard NSAIDs (at least most of the time).

Prostaglandins play a large role in important activities that are necessary for preventing the stomach from being eroded by gastric acid. In the stomach, prostaglandins:

- **Regulate mucus production.** Prostaglandins regulate the secretion of mucin and surface-active phospholipids (the substances of which mucus is composed).

- **Regulate bicarbonate production.** Bicarbonates protect the stomach wall by neutralizing stomach acid.

- **Inhibit the secretion of hydrochloric acid.** Prostaglandins play a role in the stomach's production of hydrochloric acid. This harsh substance breaks down food in the stomach, but excess acid can harm the stomach lining.

- **Increase the flow of blood to the stomach.** Prostaglandins dilate blood vessels and increase blood flow. Blood flow to the stomach is necessary for cell renewal and repair as well as carrying away acids that penetrate the stomach lining.

By interfering with prostaglandin production, NSAIDs compromise all these mucosal defense mechanisms. The result is a mucus gel that is poorly suited to defending the stomach against gastric acid. In addition, NSAIDs, especially aspirin, thin the blood by decreasing the aggregation of platelets. Indeed, many people take aspirin to prevent blood clots, heart attacks, and strokes. However, patients who take NSAIDs and develop ulcers bleed more easily and suffer from prolonged bleeding times because their blood is thinner.

How Useful Are Enteric-Coated NSAIDs?

An enteric-coated aspirin or NSAID may reduce the topical damage to your stomach, but whether that extra protection actually amounts to anything in regard to stomach health is a subject of debate. Most studies show that enteric-coated NSAIDs have little value in protecting the stomach against ulcers. Why? Because most of the damage from NSAIDs is systemic, not topical.

Enteric-coated drugs are designed to pass unaltered through the stomach and disintegrate in the intestines. Because topical damage to the stomach is not a major cause of NSAID-induced ulcers, enteric-coated NSAIDs do not show a significant improvement over other NSAIDs. They cause stomach ulcers at the same rate as other NSAIDs. This is because they interfere with prostaglandin production to the same degree as NSAIDs that are not enteric-coated.

Patients with especially sensitive stomachs may gain some advantage by taking enteric-coated NSAIDs, but taking an enteric-coated NSAID does not disqualify anyone from getting a stomach ulcer. Except for being easier to swallow, enteric-coating aspirin has no significant advantages over other aspirin.

WHO'S MOST AT RISK WHEN TAKING NSAIDS?

Assessing the risk of getting an ulcer from taking NSAIDs is problematic because studies vary as to what constitutes an ulcer, test with different NSAIDs at different dosages, and tend to focus on people over the age of 60. By strict definition, an ulcer is any erosive lesion that penetrates the mucosal lining of the stomach. To be considered an ulcer, the lesion must be three millimeters or wider in some studies, or as much as five millimeters or wider in others. Obviously, studies that use the three-millimeter-wide definition report higher incidences of ulcers.

Some NSAIDs, moreover, damage the mucosal defense more than others, as I explained earlier in this chapter (see "Assessing the Risk of Different NSAIDs" on page 57). Because different NSAIDs at different dosages are used in the studies, reaching a general-purpose conclusion about NSAIDs' risk factors is difficult.

And, compounding the problem even more, the majority of people tested in the studies are senior citizens, the group deemed most likely to get ulcers. Yet, people in this group often take other drugs besides NSAIDs and are more susceptible to ulcers to begin with because they are more likely to be infected with the *H. pylori* bacterium.

In spite of the complexities, physicians have identified several factors that increase a patient's risk of getting an ulcer from taking NSAIDs. These risk factors are discussed below.

Advanced Age

The elderly take NSAIDs more frequently than other groups because they suffer from rheumatic diseases in higher numbers. For that reason, the majority of NSAID users who develop ulcers are 60 years or older. Still, whether the elderly per se are more susceptible to ulcers or it only seems that way because they get ulcers in higher numbers, is a question worth pursuing. Most physicians believe that the elderly are more susceptible to ulcers because their immune system and mechanisms for stomach repair are weaker.

Previous History of Peptic Ulcers

Studies show that patients with a previous history of peptic ulcers or gastrointestinal bleeding are as much as fourteen times more likely to acquire an ulcer from taking NSAIDs. Patients are especially at risk during the first three months of NSAID therapy. During this period, the risk of hemorrhaging and other major complications is especially high. Doctors should be extremely careful when prescribing NSAIDs to patients with a history of peptic ulcers and gastrointestinal bleeding. Prophylactic anti-ulcer therapy—for example, the use of misoprostol (Cytotec) or another synthetic prostaglandin—is recommended for these patients.

Dosage

NSAID damage to the stomach lining is dose-dependent. The higher the dose, the more likely the patient is to get an ulcer. Still, regardless of the dose, all NSAIDs at the very least cause microscopic damage to the stomach's mucosal layer. The worst offend er is aspirin. Studies measuring the protective effect of aspirin against heart attacks invariably demonstrate as well the harmful effects of aspirin to the gastrointestinal tract. For example, in a randomized, double-blind, placebo-controlled study to determine whether low doses of aspirin (325 mg daily) decrease deaths from heart attack, researchers had 22,071 participants take aspirin on average for 60.2 months. There was a 44 percent reduction in myocardial infarction, but, at the same time, 3.6 percent of the subjects had symptoms of melena (blood in the stool) or hematemesis (the vomiting of blood). Even at low doses, aspirin poses a risk for getting an ulcer if it is taken over long periods of time.

NSAIDs and *Helicobacter Pylori*

On the surface, it would seem that peptic ulcers are more likely to occur in NSAID users who are infected with the *Helicobacter pylori* (*H. pylori*) bacterium, seeing as NSAIDs and *H. pylori* both cause peptic ulcers (Chapter 2 examines *H. pylori*). However, whether the bacterium and the drug are independent risk factors or additive risk factors is unclear. In some studies, *H. pylori* is identified as a peptic-ulcer risk factor to people who take NSAIDs; other studies conclude that being infected with *H. pylori* does not make an NSAID user more or less likely to get an ulcer. A very interesting, although not necessarily credible, theory about *H. pylori* infection and NSAIDs holds that the way in which the two work actually cancel each other out:

• Prostaglandin levels in the stomach increase at the site of an *H. pylori* infection. This has the effect of balancing out the NSAID, which normally inhibits the production of prostaglandins.

• NSAIDs increase the stomach's production of hydrochloric acid. More acid in the stomach means that fewer bacteria, *H. pylori* included, survive.

• *H. pylori* bacteria hide in the defensive mucus layer on the lining of the stomach. By eroding this mucus layer, NSAIDs give *H. pylori* bacteria fewer places to hide.

Evidence shows that the bleeding and perforation that accompany NSAID-caused ulcers is usually more severe than the bleeding and perforation that accompany ulcers caused by an *H. pylori* infection. Why this is so might have something to do with NSAIDs' blood-thinning properties. NSAIDs are anti-coagulators; they make blood clots less likely to occur, but they encourage more bleeding.

NSAIDs and Steroids

Steroids—the word is short for the scientific term for the drugs, *corticosteroids*—are synthetic derivatives of a natural steroid called cortisol, which is produced by the adrenal glands. Steroids suppress the immune system. Doctors prescribe prednisone, cortisone, hydrocortisone, and other steroids to fight inflammation in injured or damaged tissue. Steroids are used to treat rheumatoid arthritis, asthma, lupus, myositis (muscle inflammation), and systemic vasculitis (inflammation of the blood vessels). They are used to prevent transplanted organs from being rejected. Often, steroids are injected into joints to treat arthritis and other inflammatory illnesses.

In contrast to NSAIDs, which work by inhibiting the body's production of prostaglandins, steroids work by slowing the release and activity of white blood cells and other chemicals associated with the immune system.

Most physicians are under the impression that taking steroids, like taking NSAIDs, can cause peptic ulcers, but studies have produced conflicting conclusions. In an analysis of ninety-three studies involving the administration of steroids, H.O. Conn et al. concluded, "Peptic ulcer is a rare complication of corticosteroid therapy." But J. Messer et al., in an analysis of seventy-one clinical trials, found that "corticosteroids do increase the risk of peptic ulcers and gastrointestinal hemorrhage." The problem with assessing whether steroids cause peptic ulcers is that the patients under study are often very ill and are usually taking several medications at once. Determining which drug is responsible for causing the ulcer becomes a matter of speculation. What is certain, however, is that taking NSAIDs and steroids at the same time greatly increases a patient's chances of getting a peptic ulcer.

By the way, the corticoid steroids discussed here are different from the anabolic steroids that foolhardy bodybuilders and athletes take. Anabolic steroids are synthetic drugs related to male sex hormones. They were developed in the 1930s to treat hypogonadism, a condition in which the testicles do not produce enough testosterone for normal adolescent growth. Athletes take anabolic steroids to promote the development and healing of skeletal muscle tissue. However, the prolonged use of anabolic steroids can cause water retention, acne, high blood pressure, liver damage, impotence, balding, kidney problems, and gynecomastia (the formation of female breasts on men). People who take anabolic steroids are also susceptible to "roid rage," a psychotic condition in which the subject demonstrates extraordinary anger and a propensity for violence.

SYMPTOMS OF NSAID-CAUSED ULCERS

One of the most disturbing aspects of NSAID-related ulcer disease is the unexpectedness with which the disease appears. In ulcers caused by *H. pylori* bacterial infections, patients usually experience gastritis, bloating, and abdominal pain before the onset of the ulcer. These symptoms alert patients that something is wrong and should encourage them to visit a doctor. In the case of an NSAID-caused ulcer, however, the ulcer can appear without any warning signs. Sometimes internal bleeding is the first symptom. Often, patients don't realize that they have an ulcer until it is well advanced and therefore difficult to treat.

Roughly half the people who take NSAIDs for long periods of time experience dyspepsia—nausea, nonspecific pain, discomfort, and bloating in the upper abdominal region just below the rib cage. Of the NSAID users who complain of dyspepsia, however, the majority will not acquire an ulcer. Dyspepsia is common in the first month of therapy and usually disappears over time. Dyspepsia, therefore, cannot be considered a reliable symptom of a peptic ulcer caused by NSAIDs.

The fact is, people who have NSAID-caused ulcers are less likely than others to have symptoms of any kind. As many as 60 percent of patients who take NSAIDs and have bleeding ulcers show no symptoms until the bleeding occurs. In ulcer patients who aren't taking NSAIDs, only 25 percent lack symptoms until their ulcers start bleeding.

NSAIDS AS THE CAUSE OF OTHER DISEASES

Besides raising your risk of getting an ulcer, NSAIDs can cause other diseases and health complications. These pages look at some side effects of taking NSAIDs—kidney diseases, liver diseases, miscarriage, and infertility. Taking the occasional NSAID poses very little health risk, but people who take NSAIDs for long periods of time run the risk of getting an ulcer or one of the diseases or conditions described below.

Kidney (Renal) Disease

You have two kidneys, each about the size of a fist. Kidneys perform many tasks that are important for good health. Among other things, they release hormones that regulate blood pressure and control the production of red blood cells. Approximately one-fifth of the blood that is pumped from the heart goes to the kidneys. There, blood is cleansed as it passes through millions of tiny filters called the glomeruli. Cleansed blood then returns to the bloodstream. The waste material filtered from the blood—excess water, dying cells, drugs, and other debris—is sent through ducts called tubules to the bladder, where, eventually, it passes out of the body in the urine.

Most of the damage that NSAIDs do to the kidneys involves blood flow to the glomeruli and tubules, the filtering units of the kidneys. It appears that prostaglandins play a role in dilating blood vessels and permitting blood to pass to these filtering units. Because NSAIDs inhibit prostaglandin production (and prostaglandins are necessary for the glomeruli to do their work), the prolonged use of NSAIDs can lead to kidney disease and kidney failure. Blood is not filtered at the proper rate and urine output decreases. As a result, toxic waste cannot exit the body and concentrates in the bloodstream.

A single glomerulus and its tubule are called a nephron. Kidney diseases caused by NSAIDs fall in the nephritis category, and are as follows:

- **Nephrotic syndrome.** Condition in which damaged kidneys allow large amounts of protein to leak from the blood into the urine. Because protein helps to keep fluid in the bloodstream, the lack of protein permits fluid to leave the bloodstream and enter tissue. This causes tissue to swell, especially in the legs and the area under the eyes, in a condition known as edema.

- **Analgesic nephropathy.** The name for nephritis caused by the prolonged use of NSAIDs and other over-the-counter pain remedies.

- **Interstitial nephritis (also called tubulointerstitial nephritis).** This disease is caused by inflammation of the tubules, the ducts through which waste matter passes out of the glomeruli. Symptoms include a decrease in urine output and kidney failure.

People who take NSAIDs and have pre-existing kidney conditions or high blood pressure are especially susceptible to kidney failure. Fortunately, simple blood tests are available for measuring the amount of waste products in blood that are normally removed by the kidneys. If you are concerned about NSAIDs causing damage to your kidneys, ask your doctor about the Serum Creatinine level or BUN (blood urine nitrogen) blood test. These tests show whether the kidneys are properly removing waste products from the blood.

Hepatic (Liver) Diseases

Overall, incidences of NSAIDs damaging the liver are rare, but a recent study of hepatitis C patients taking NSAIDs raised eyebrows in the medical community. In the study conducted at the Pennsylvania State University College of Medicine, researchers looked at three patients with hepatitis C who took the NSAID ibuprofen (Motrin, Advil). In all three patients, the liver enzymes AST and ALT increased fivefold after taking the drug. Normally, these aminotransferase enzymes reside in liver cells, but they are released into the bloodstream when the liver is damaged. Doctors measure AST and ALT levels in the blood to determine the extent of the liver damage. When all three patients stopped taking ibuprofen, their AST and ALT enzyme levels decreased markedly.

Interestingly, the authors of this study recommended giving hepatitis C patients acetaminophen (Tylenol, Exdol, Panadol, Paracetamol) instead of NSAIDs. However, in large doses, especially if alcohol is taken along with the drug, acetaminophen can cause severe liver damage. If you are taking acetaminophen and you are an adult, don't exceed the recommended dosage of 4,000 mg (eight extra-strength pills) over twenty-four hours. If you drink more than two alcoholic beverages a day, don't take more than 2,000 mg daily of the drug.

Children and teenagers who have upper respiratory illnesses, chickenpox, or influenza should avoid aspirin because they run the risk of developing Reye's syndrome. This rare disease leads to swelling of the brain, fat accumulation in the liver, and, eventually, liver failure. What causes Reye's syndrome is unclear, but scientists have established a link between the syndrome and taking aspirin for viral illnesses. Symptoms include vomiting and nausea.

Miscarriage

Taking NSAIDs may increase the risk of miscarriage. A study of 1,063 pregnant women in the San Francisco Bay Area found that the risk of miscarriage is 80 percent higher in women who take NSAIDs. In the study, 149 miscarriages occurred among the 980 women who did not take NSAIDS, for a miscarriage rate of 15 percent; but among the fifty-three women who did take the drugs, thirteen women miscarried for a miscarriage rate of 24.5 percent. Researchers reported that the risk of miscarrying was highest when women took NSAIDs around the time of conception or when they took the drugs for more than a week.

A study conducted in Denmark produced similar results. That study compared 1,462 pregnant women who had prescriptions for NSAIDs to 17,259 pregnant women who did not take NSAIDs. It found that taking NSAIDs increased the risk of miscarriage (but not the risk of birth defects or premature births). To be fair, critics of these studies point out that many of the women who miscarried may have taken an NSAID to treat the abdominal pain resulting from miscarriage itself. In other words, these women may have taken an NSAID after they began to miscarry, in which case NSAIDs were not to blame for their miscarriages.

Infertility and Anovulation

A handful of studies indicate that taking NSAIDs can cause infertility in women. Specifically, the drugs can cause luteinizing unruptured follicle syndrome (LUFS), a condition in which follicles in the ovaries fail to release eggs and patients are infertile. The reason why NSAIDs affect the release of eggs from the ovaries is unclear, but it appears that the release of eggs has something to do with prostaglandins. As explained earlier in this chapter, NSAIDs hinder prostaglandin production in the body.

CONCLUSION

Whenever you take a drug, you have to weigh the benefits against the risks. In the case of NSAIDs, the risks are formidable. People who take NSAIDs for a long period of time may develop peptic ulcers, suffer from kidney and liver diseases, or have a miscarriage. To people who are afflicted with rheumatoid arthritis or osteoporosis, running the risks of taking NSAIDs is worthwhile. For these people, the long-term use of NSAIDs is necessary to live a normal life without crippling pain.

While COX-2 inhibitors may have some benefits to people who must take NSAIDs, this class of NSAID will need to be refined or improved if COX-2s are to be a viable alternative to standard NSAIDs. It appears, for the time being, that the harmful side effects of NSAIDs will remain with us. Doctors concerned for the stomach health of their patients who must take NSAIDs may consider the addition of natural products such as Zinc-Carnosine. Zinc-Carnosine is something of a preventative medicine in that it can strengthen the stomach mucosa against the corrosive effect of NSAIDs. I will explain the benefits of Zinc-Carnosine in detail in Chapter 8.

4

Lifestyle Causes and Factors

hile medical research has uncovered two major causes of peptic ulcers—*H. pylori* and NSAIDs—there are, unfortunately, a number of other causes that also contribute to this condition. Undetected, these other factors lead to the same painful and unhealthy state. In this chapter, I will discuss genetic predisposition, smoking, alcohol, diet, stress, and various medical procedures and rare conditions that can cause ulcers.

The funny thing is that not so long ago, these "other" causes and factors were considered the primary causes of peptic ulcer disease. The discovery of *H. pylori* changed this idea, allowing an all-too-willing public to think of ulcers as finally being under control. The fact is, however, that the causes described in this chapter are as potent as *H. pylori* and NSAIDs in creating the right conditions necessary for this disease.

A COMING TOGETHER OF FACTORS?

It seems the more one learns about ulcers, the deeper the mystery becomes. Conventional wisdom says that *H. pylori* infections cause 75 percent of stomach ulcers and 90 percent of duodenal ulcers, and the rest are caused by non-steroidal anti-inflammatory drugs (NSAIDs). However, other culprits besides *H. pylori* and NSAIDs undoubtedly help to cause ulcers. An interesting study conducted in Rochester, New York, of ulcer patients who did not take NSAIDs found that only 61 percent of patients were infected with *H. pylori*.

71

How did the other 39 percent of patients acquire an ulcer, given that they didn't take NSAIDs and weren't infected by the *H. pylori* bacterium?

In a similar study conducted in Orlando, Florida, of ulcer patients who did not take NSAIDs, only 27 percent were infected with *H. pylori*. Studies like these have called into question whether other factors besides *H. pylori* and NSAIDs play an important role in the formation of peptic ulcers. Is the role of *H. pylori* infection being overestimated? After all, most people who are infected with *H. pylori* do not develop ulcers. Could it be, in people who are infected, that *H. pylori* is being blamed for causing ulcers when the blame should rightly be attributed as well to other factors or causes? As I have discussed, the gastrointestinal tract is an extremely complex environment. It could be that ulcers are caused by a coming together of different factors—not a single one.

THE GENETIC COMPONENT

It used to be considered ultimate truth that ulcers run in families and certain people have a genetic predisposition to getting peptic ulcers. Some evidence points to the conclusion that there is a genetic component in the formation of ulcers:

- In studies done on identical twins, in 50 percent of cases, if one twin had an ulcer, so did the other.

- The parents, siblings, and children of people with ulcers are three times more likely to have an ulcer themselves.

- People with blood type O are 35 percent more likely to get a duodenal ulcer, according to one study. The reason is that *H. pylori* bacteria are better able to attach to the intestinal mucus layer of people in blood group O.

- Men who do not secrete ABO blood group antigens in their saliva are twice as likely to be infected with *H. pylori* bacteria, and twice as likely to get ulcers.

Studies have shown that people who smoke and abuse alcohol have a genetic predisposition toward this kind of behavior. Many alcoholics almost certainly have a genetic predisposition to alcoholism. It could be that ulcers have a genetic component in so far as people who are predisposed to abuse alcohol and cigarettes are more likely to get ulcers because they expose themselves to more risks.

On the other hand, it could be that ulcers don't so much run in families as they cluster in families. The discovery of *H. pylori* as a cause of peptic ulcers (see Chapter 2) threw a wrench into the genetic predisposition argument. Families share the same germs as well as the same genes. Perhaps ulcers run in families because family members spread the same bacteria and viruses to one another. *H. pylori* can infect infants but not cause a peptic disease or full-blown ulcer for decades, so even an ulcer that occurs late in life can be the result of family members sharing *H. pylori* bacteria years ago.

SMOKING

Statistics show very clearly that smokers are more likely to develop ulcers, especially ulcers of the duodenum, than nonsmokers. Smokers are actually twice as likely to develop ulcers as nonsmokers. In one study, the likelihood of ulcer perforation was ten times higher in smokers than nonsmokers. A 1989 report issued by the Surgeon General of the United States declared that ulcers are more prevalent, slower to heal, and more likely to cause death in smokers than nonsmokers.

Why people who smoke get ulcers more frequently than nonsmokers is a subject of debate. Scientists have advanced many different reasons:

- **Smoking increases the amount of acid secreted by the stomach.** This higher production of acid irritates the stomach lining and leads to an ulcer.

- **Smoking increases the risk of being infected with the *H. pylori* bacterium.** This could have something to do with the harmful effects of smoking on the immune system and the oxidation that accompanies smoking. A study conducted at the Prince of Wales Hospital at the Chinese University of Hong Kong found that a smoker's risk of getting a recurring ulcer is roughly the same as a nonsmoker's after *H. pylori* has been erad-icated. In the study, researchers tracked eighty-three smoking and two-hundred-four nonsmoking ulcer patients who had been treated for *H. pylori* infections. The percentage of patients who had reoccurring ulcers in both groups was roughly the same. This suggests that smoking in combination with an *H. pylori* infection, not smoking alone, is the reason why smokers are more likely to get an ulcer.

- **Smoking reduces the pancreas's production of sodium bicar-bonate.** This alkali neutralizes gastric acid as it passes from the stomach to the duodenum. Because sodium bicarbonate is pro-duced in lower amounts, gastric acid from the stomach can find its way into the duodenum and cause ulcers there.

- **Smoking decreases the flow of blood to the stomach.** This blood flow is necessary for carrying away debris and acids that penetrate the stomach lining, for cell renewal, and for cell repair.

- **Smoking slows the emptying of the gastrointestinal tract.** Mat-ter pushed from the stomach into the duodenum remains there longer, where it may backtrack into the stomach to irritate the stomach lining.

Add all of these factors together, and it isn't hard to see how smoking increases your chances of getting an ulcer.

ALCOHOL

Alcohol's relationship to ulcers is not clearly understood. People who drink high alcohol-content liquor or who are alcoholics are more likely to get peptic ulcers. At one time, it was thought that this was so because alcohol increases stomach acidity. Paradoxi-cally, however, studies show that drinking alcoholic beverages at concentrations of 5 percent (10 proof) or lower stimulates the secre-tion of gastric acid, but drinking liquor with alcohol concentrations above 10 percent (20 proof) actually diminishes acid secretion in the stomach.

Why, then, is drinking alcoholic beverages associated with peptic ulcer disease? One reason could have to do with a genetic predisposition. People who are genetically predisposed to drink alcohol irresponsibly are also predisposed to undertaking other unsafe behaviors that put them at risk for getting an ulcer. Drinking alcohol on an empty stomach almost certainly increases your chances of getting an ulcer. Food buffers the stomach wall and protects it from irritation by alcohol. Alcohol concentration is another factor. Drinking wine, beer, cider or another low-concentration alcoholic beverage, especially if it is taken with lunch or dinner, does not significantly increase your chances of getting an ulcer, but drinking strong liquor on an empty stomach puts you at a greater risk.

I am skeptical of those who counsel people never to drink alcohol for the sake of their health. Having a drink now and then is pleasurable, and experiencing pleasure in life is one of the best defenses against disease. Studies show conclusively that people who are depressed are more likely to get sick than people who are content. If drinking modest amounts of alcohol makes you content, the health benefits you get from your glass of wine or beer far outweigh the risk you run of getting a peptic ulcer.

DIET

The notion that you can cure diseases with diet is as old as humankind. As a physician, however, I have to ask myself if curing patients by urging them to eat a certain diet is practical. Studies show that people's taste in food is formed in the first six years of life, and, indeed, predilections for certain foods may be written into our genes. For those reasons, most people cannot, practically speaking, change their diet a great deal. Tragically, I saw this firsthand when I was a youngster in Swiss refugee camps during World War II. Most people will only eat what they have been culturally and genetically programmed to eat—that is, what they have been culturally and genetically programmed to enjoy. In the refugee camps, I saw people die of self-inflicted hunger because they couldn't bring themselves to eat the foul gruel that was our daily pittance.

Any diet, no matter what its purpose, has to start with the premise that people in the long run will eat only what they enjoy.

Alcohol as a Bactericidal

Drinking alcoholic beverages, in one regard, helps to prevent stomach ulcers because alcohol, an antibacterial agent, kills the *H. pylori* bacterium. Consider the following studies:

- In a study conducted in England, researchers looked at the drinking habits of 4,902 individuals, 1,634 of whom were infected with *H. pylori*. They discovered that the risk of being infected with *H. pylori* in people who drank three to six glasses of wine per week was 11 percent lower than the risk to people who did not drink wine. The risk to individuals in the study who drank more than six glasses of wine per week was 17 percent lower. This being England, the study included subjects who drank beer, and they, too, showed a reduced risk for being infected by *H. pylori*. The authors of the study wrote, "Our data indicate that modest consumption of beer or wine—approximately one drink per day per week—protects against active *H. pylori* infection, presumably by facilitating eradication of the organisms. However, the data do not enable us to comment on the relevance of patterns of wine and beer consumption."

- In another study conducted in Spain, researchers looked at the drinking habits of people who had been given triple eradication therapy (omeprazole, clarithromycin, and amoxicillin), the conventional treatment for an *H. pylori* infection, to find out how alcohol consumption helped or hindered the elimination of *H. pylori*. More so than other factors—smoking status, sex, age, length of illness—what determined whether *H. pylori* was eradicated in a subject was his or her consumption of alcohol. *H. pylori* was eradicated in 70 percent of people who didn't drink wine, but 79 percent of people who drank at least two glasses of wine each day and 100 percent of people who drank more than two glasses of wine daily successfully rid themselves of their *H. pylori* infections.

Wine has a long history of being a medicine, so it should not be a surprise that wine is effective against *H. pylori* bacteria. For example, British soldiers in India drank claret as "a sovereign preventative against the prevalent cholera." In 1892, after contaminating water with cholera bacteria, Dr. Alois Pick diluted the water with wine and drank the mixture. He lived to tell the tale, proving once and for all that wine is bactericidal.

People are unwilling to be force-fed. This simple premise was very well illustrated by the failure of anti-ulcer diets in the first half of the last century. For fifty years, the conventional thinking was that ulcers are caused by eating spicy foods, citrus fruit, coffee, and other foods that fall in the tangy or sharp category. Patients were made to eat the opposite of spicy food—they ate malted milk, porridge, whey, and other bland food to settle their stomachs. Knowing what we know today about the causes of ulcers, it is painful to imagine ulcer patients living on these bland diets for years at a time without being cured. This passage from a 1907 medical text describes a typical treatment for gastric ulcers in early twentieth-century America. It comes from *The Eclectic Practice of Medicine* (1907 edition), a popular physician's manual written by Dr. Rolla L. Thomas.

[Ulcer] Treatment.—In the earlier stages the treatment will be similar to that for gastritis, which it so closely resembles; but as soon as the symptoms are sufficiently pronounced to warrant a diagnosis, the patient must be put to bed and kept absolutely quiet. He must be given to understand that a cure means from four to six months in bed. Nothing will take the place of rest in the recumbent position. The diet must receive particular attention, for the most skillful line of medication will fail if we neglect this phase of the treatment. Only the blandest and most easily digested food should be allowed, peptonized foods being among the best. Where there is great irritability of the stomach and vomiting, the stomach should have absolute rest, nourishment being given by the rectum. As soon, however, as the stomach will tolerate food, I prefer giving it by mouth.

Pepsin whey is one of the blandest and most kindly received foods that can be given; malted milk, Eskay's food [a kind of baby food], and Wells, Richardson Co.'s cereal milk are also well received. It is a good plan to change the food every two or three days, so that the patient will not tire of any one food. Where the stomach is in a rebellious mood, albumen water [water mixed with egg whites] is generally well received. The white of one egg, stirred in a half glass of water, and taken at one time, or, in smaller quantities, one or two hours being consumed in the taking, will be found helpful.

Some spicy foods increase acid production and aggravate ulcers. Coffee can weaken the esophageal sphincter, permitting stomach acid to rise into the esophagus and cause heartburn. Dairy products such as milk, cream, and ice cream were commonly recommended for ulcers, but we know today that milk and other dairy products do nothing but antagonize ulcers. In the short term, milk relieves ulcer pain by coating the stomach lining and temporarily neutralizing gastric acid. In the long run, however, the calcium and protein in milk stimulate gastric acid production, and this excess gastric acid causes more pain and suffering for the ulcer patient.

As far as healing or relieving ulcer pain with a diet is concerned, the best thing patients can do is moderate their diets and learn to be aware of which foods cause them gastric discomfort or gastric pain. A patient who is willing to monitor his or her diet this way will eventually come around to a diet that relieves ulcer pain and perhaps helps cure ulcers. Anybody who believes that a significant number of ulcers can be cured by a strict eating regimen is not taking human nature into account. People want to eat what they enjoy. This is nothing less than a matter of physiology.

STRESS

While stress isn't a primary cause of ulcers, as physicians used to believe, stress undoubtedly plays a role. No organ reacts to and resonates stress more acutely than the stomach. After all, you can turn your stomach, have butterflies in your stomach, have an awful feeling in the pit of your stomach, and, if you are immune to stress, have a cast-iron stomach. Stress engages the nervous system, the cardiovascular system, and hormone production. When you experience stress, your adrenal glands secrete hormones, your sympathetic nervous system becomes quickly aroused, your heart beats faster, your blood pressure rises, and the amount of sugar in your blood increases. Sustained periods of stress can tax the nervous system and cardiovascular system. Stress can disrupt hormone production. Long-term stress can lead to cardiovascular disease, fatigue, and depression. The cumulative effect of all this may result in a weakened immune system—and, therefore, a stomach and duodenum that are more susceptible to bacterial infection leading to ulceration.

Numerous studies have been undertaken to measure the influence of stress on the formation of ulcers. The problem with these studies is that "stress" and "stressors" are hard to define. What is stressful to one person may get a shrug from someone else. Anger, anxiety, depression—the typical manifestations of stress—are hard to measure. Compounding this problem even further, stress can be a consequence of ulcer disease. In some patients, the ulcer may precede the stress, not the stress the ulcer.

We do know that extreme stress can cause ulcers. For experimental purposes in the laboratory, scientists can induce multiple bleeding ulcers in rats by immobilizing them—essentially by tying them down—for two to three hours. After air raids during the London blitz, hospitals in London reported increases in patients with perforated ulcers. Many people in World War II concentration camps died of bleeding ulcers. Critically ill patients brought into the intensive care unit with severe injuries—especially respiratory failure, blood clots, head trauma, or severe burns—may quickly develop acute gastric ulcers, a condition called *acute hemorrhagic gastropathy.* Doctors speculate that excessive gastric secretion and a weakening of the mucosal barrier that guards the stomach against gastric acid causes these ulcers.

At any rate, the "ulcer personality" of medical literature prior to the discovery of *H. pylori* has packed his bags and left town forever. It used to be thought that highly driven, aggressive, type-A personalities were more susceptible to ulcers, but we know that the meek and mild get ulcers at the same rate as the hostile and the antagonistic (in my experience, aggressive type-A personalities give ulcers more frequently than they get them).

OTHER CAUSES

In addition to genetic and lifestyle factors, there are a number of medical procedures and rare conditions that can cause peptic ulcers—Zollinger-Ellison syndrome, Meckel's diverticulum, Barrett's esophagus, and gastroenterostomies. While relatively few in number, these other causes should be considered in cases that rule out all the other factors already discussed in this book.

Zollinger-Ellison Syndrome

A small number of tumors (between 0.1 and 1 percent) are caused by Zollinger-Ellison syndrome. This syndrome causes the stomach to produce excessive amounts of hydrochloric acid. Normally, when food arrives in the stomach, cells in the stomach secrete gastrin into the blood. This hormone, in turn, stimulates the production of hydrochloric acid in the stomach so that the recently arrived food can be broken down and assimilated. As acid levels in the stomach rise, gastrin secretion in the stomach gradually ceases. In this way, the stomach always has the right amount of acid to digest food.

In patients with Zollinger-Ellison syndrome, a malignant tumor called a *gastrinoma* in the pancreas, duodenum, or bile ducts, produces gastrin hormones. As a result, the bloodstream is flooded with gastrin, and this causes a markedly higher production of hydrochloric acid in the stomach. People with Zollinger-Ellison syndrome develop recurring ulcers due to this excessive acid. Treatments include proton pump inhibitors to control the excessive production of stomach acid, and, in some cases, surgery to partially or completely remove the gastrinoma.

Meckel's Diverticulum

Meckel's diverticulum is a small pouch or sac in the wall of the small intestine near the point where the small and large intestines meet. This pouch is made of the same kind of tissue found in the stomach, as opposed to the small intestine. As such, it produces stomach acid, and this acid can cause irritation or an ulcer. If the ulcer perforates, waste products can leak into the abdomen and cause peritonitis. The diverticulum can also cause a blockage in the small intestine.

Meckel's diverticulum is the most common congenital anomaly of the gastrointestinal tract. It is present in 2 percent of newborns, but most people never show any symptoms or have any problems. The pouch is the remnant of the duct that connects the developing embryo to the yolk sac. In most people, the duct disappears, but if it fails to do so, it remains as a Meckel's diverticulum, named for Johann F. Meckel, the German anatomist who first described it.

Barrett's Esophagus

About one in ten patients with gastroesophageal reflux disease (GERD) develop a condition called Barrett's esophagus. GERD is nothing less than persistent, chronic heartburn. It is caused by gastric acid refluxing—or splashing upward—into the esophagus, the ten-inch-long muscular tube that connects the throat to the stomach. The cells that line the esophagus are not equipped to handle harsh gastric acid from the stomach. In Barrett's esophagus, cells like the kind that line the stomach grow in the esophagus as a defense mechanism against gastric acid. However, being stomach-like mucosal cells, the cells secrete acid. This can cause what amounts to a peptic ulcer in the esophagus.

Gastroenterostomy

A gastroenterostomy is a surgical procedure in which a cancerous growth in the duodenum, the first portion of the small intestine, is removed and the stomach is surgically connected to the jejunum, the second portion of the small intestine. After the surgery, the jejunum is exposed to gastric acid that would normally be neutralized in the duodenum. This can result in ulcers in the jejunum.

CONCLUSION

Where once medical science had clearly focused on stress and diet as the leading causes of peptic ulcers, today it is difficult for researchers to qualify or quantify the part that lifestyle factors actually play. However, as we have seen, lifestyle factors do play a role in the development of peptic ulcers. From a genetic predisposition to alcohol abuse to stress, each factor weakens the body's ability to keep itself in balance and protect itself from getting peptic ulcers and other diseases.

The key point to remember here is that lifestyles can be changed for the better. While it may not be easy, modifying one or more of our behaviors can influence the odds of getting an ulcer. And while maintaining a high level of health may not guarantee an ulcer-free existence, it does allow you to become part of a long-term solution.

5

Symptoms
and Diagnoses

When I was in medical school a number of years ago, we learned very simple techniques for diagnosing peptic ulcers. Patients with ulcers, we were told, experience pain two to five hours after eating, as well as pain at night. A patient who goes to bed at ten o'clock will wake up between midnight and three o'clock with stomach pain. We learned that abdominal tenderness was a sign of a peptic ulcer. We were taught how to physically examine a patient's epigastrium—the upper third of the abdomen, directly below the diaphragm—for signs of tenderness. In those days you could X-ray a patient's stomach and duodenum for signs of an ulcer, but understanding the severity of a patient's ulcer by examining those unsophisticated X-rays made for a crude diagnosis.

Medical science has come a long way in the past fifty years in its ability to recognize ulcer symptoms and test for the presence of an ulcer. This chapter should enable you to clearly recognize the most common symptoms of an ulcer. It will then explain the various tests that doctors use to determine whether or not an ulcer is present. By chapter's end, you will know what tests and procedures may lie ahead. With this information, you will be in a better position to understand your options and work with your doctor.

SYMPTOMS OF A PEPTIC ULCER

Unless an ulcer proves severe and starts hemorrhaging, reading the symptoms of an ulcer can be difficult. Population-based studies of peptic ulcer disease rates show that 4 percent of patients have no symptoms at all. Uncomplicated ulcer disease shares many symptoms with dyspepsia, as well as other gastrointestinal diseases. Symptoms vary from patient to patient and are not present all the time. Some patients can tolerate pain better than others; some patients exaggerate their symptoms. The upshot of all this is, short of diagnostic testing (a subject taken up later in this chapter), knowing for certain whether someone has an ulcer can be difficult. These pages look at the most common symptoms of ulcer disease—the general symptoms as well as the more specific ones.

Abdominal Pain

Typically, people with ulcers experience a gnawing or burning pain in the epigastric region of the abdomen, the area in the upper third of the abdomen between the navel and the breastbone. However, pain in this area can also be caused by a host of other gastric problems such as heartburn, reflux disease (GERD), pancreatitis, and gastric and pancreatic cancer. Moreover, ulcers caused by taking NSAIDs can appear suddenly without any warning pain, perhaps because NSAIDs are pain-relievers and they obscure the pain of having an ulcer.

Two-thirds of patients with a duodenal ulcer and one-third of patients with a stomach ulcer wake up between midnight and three o'clock with sharp pain in their abdomens. However, this pain is also present in a third of patients with non-ulcer dyspepsia.

Dyspepsia

Most people who get an ulcer experience some degree of stomach upset referred to as dyspepsia. However, fewer than 30 percent of the people diagnosed with dyspepsia who undergo an endoscopy develop an ulcer. And to complicate matters even further, doctors do not all agree on how to define this elusive disease. The symptoms of dyspepsia are too subjective and open to interpretation. In 30 to 60 percent of patients, doctors cannot determine a cause for dyspepsia.

Dyspepsia—the word comes from the Greek *dys*, for "bad," and *peptein*, for "digestion"—is a persistent or recurring pain or discomfort located in the upper abdomen. According to one study, 15 percent of Americans experience dyspepsia annually, although most do not seek medical care. Symptoms can include abdominal bloating and a feeling of fullness, nausea, heartburn, belching, and, in severe cases, vomiting. To be considered chronic, symptoms must be present for three months. Dyspepsia can accompany the use of antibiotics and other drugs, gastroesophageal reflux disease (GERD), irritable bowel syndrome, stomach cancer, gall bladder disease, liver disease, and other ailments. Sometimes, in a condition known as non-ulcer dyspepsia (or functional dyspepsia), patients experience the symptoms of dyspepsia without any identifiable cause.

To help doctors distinguish between non-ulcer dyspepsia and dyspepsia brought about by irritable bowel syndrome, GERD, or a peptic ulcer, doctors established the Rome classification system. According to this system, a patient's dyspepsia is more likely to be caused by an ulcer if the patient is experiencing acute upper abdominal pain, as well as three or more of these symptoms:

- Pain that is well localized in the epigastrium (the upper middle third of the abdomen, directly below the diaphragm).

- Pain that is relieved by eating.

- Pain that is relieved by antacids or H_2 blockers.

- Pain that occurs before meals or when the patient is hungry.

- Pain that awakens the patient from sleep.

- Pain that occurs with remissions lasting for weeks.

Frankly, dyspepsia is one of those general-purpose terms that physicians use to describe a mixed bag of symptoms ("irritable bowel syndrome" is another such term). We don't really know what causes dyspepsia or whether the condition should properly be considered a symptom rather than a disease. Stress control, exercise, meditation, and other relaxation techniques can often cure functional dyspepsia, a type of dyspepsia for which the doctor can't find any known cause.

Meal-Related Pain

Gastric ulcer pain doesn't follow a pattern, but the pain of a duodenal ulcer is usually sharpest one to three hours after eating a meal. Eating often relieves ulcer pain temporarily because food buffers the lining of the stomach and prevents ulcerated tissue from being scalded by stomach acid. Antacid tablets have a similar effect. They are effective for one to three hours, but then the pain returns.

Interrupted Sleep

The production of stomach acid is highest during sleep. For this reason, a patient who has a peptic ulcer often wakes up at night when excessive stomach acid irritates his or her ulcer. *H. pylori* may also play a part in awakening the patient. The toxins produced by *H. pylori* bacteria are felt more keenly at night when there is an absence of food in the stomach.

Symptoms Associated with a Hemorrhaging Ulcer

About 15 percent of peptic ulcer patients experience hemorrhaging. When the process of tissue ulceration damages an underlying blood vessel, the open sore bleeds into the gastrointestinal tract. Hemorrhaging is most likely to occur in people over age 60 who are taking non-steroidal anti-inflammatory drugs (NSAIDs). The anti-clotting activity of these drugs and their erosive effect on the stomach's mucosal defenses encourage bleeding. However, 10 to 20 percent of patients who hemorrhage bleed mildly and do not show any symptoms of a bleeding ulcer. The amount of blood flow has to do with whether the ulcer erodes into a major artery or a small blood vessel. Approximately 80 percent of ulcers stop bleeding without treatment. In the following discussion, I explain the symptoms of a hemorrhaging ulcer.

Bloody Stool

Blood in the stool can originate anywhere in the intestinal tract. For that reason, numerous diseases, from hemorrhoids to cancers, can cause a bloody stool. The medical term for bloody stools is *melena*.

In patients with ulcers, the stools are either very dark or black, rather than maroon or bright red in color (the blood in stools appears black because it has been digested).

For a stool to be black, approximately two tablespoons (sixty milliliters) of blood must have been lost in the gastrointestinal (GI) tract. This kind of severe bleeding occurs most frequently in the upper GI tract as the result of a tear in the esophagus, gastritis, or a peptic ulcer. Bright red blood in a stool indicates bleeding in the lower part of the GI tract, in the large intestine or rectum. This bleeding is usually caused by a fissure (rip in the skin), polyp, or hemorrhoid.

Iron supplements, blueberries, black licorice, lead poisoning, and medications containing bismuth, such as Pepto-Bismol, can also cause stools to turn black—so a black or dark stool is not necessarily the symptom of an ulcer or bleeding in the GI tract. To find out how much blood is being passed, doctors can perform a fecal occult blood test (also called a Hemoccult or stool gaiac test). Whatever the cause, you should see a doctor immediately if you notice persistent blood in your stools.

Vomiting Blood

Enough internal bleeding can cause patients to vomit blood, a condition known as *hematemesis*. If the hemorrhage is serious, partially digested blood in vomit has the appearance of coffee grounds. Vomiting blood can also be caused by prolonged retching, an inflammation of the esophagus, gastritis, or other diseases. In any event, if you are vomiting blood, it is the symptom of a major medical problem and you should seek medical care immediately.

Other Symptoms

The loss of blood that accompanies a hemorrhaging ulcer can cause low blood pressure and a rapid heart rate, because the lowered blood volume caused by blood loss requires the heart to work harder to deliver a more adequate supply of blood throughout the body. Symptoms typical of anemia—fatigue, clammy hands, pale skin, and dizziness—can occur. The decreased flow of blood to the brain can cause disorientation, confusion, and, paradoxically, insomnia. The insomnia is caused by anxiety on the part of the patient.

Common Symptoms of a Peptic Ulcer

If you are experiencing three or more of the following symptoms, it is important to seek professional medical attention.

- Pain that is relieved by eating a meal, but then returns approximately one to three hours later.

- Pain that gets worse when you eat or drink.

- Stomach pain that awakens you during the night.

- A bloated or full feeling that occurs often.

- Weight loss.

- Dark or black stools.

- The presence of blood in vomit.

A SURVEY OF DIAGNOSTIC TESTS

As often as not, patients with the classic symptoms of peptic ulcer disease actually suffer from a different gastrointestinal disorder. Because a physical examination and review of a patient's medical history are not reliable for determining whether an ulcer is present, doctors rely on diagnostic tests. Some tests look for the presence of *H. pylori* bacteria, the bacteria that can cause ulcers. Other tests permit doctors to inspect the stomach and duodenum for ulcers and, in some instances, take biopsies. In the section that follows, I will be presenting these tests, and explaining why doctors may select one test over the other. I will also be comparing the merits and reliability of these different tests. Table 5.1 on page 89 briefly describes the various diagnostic tests for peptic ulcer disease that are examined in this chapter.

PROCEDURES FOR EXAMINING THE STOMACH AND DUODENUM

The closer doctors can examine the stomach and duodenum, the better they can tell whether a patient has a peptic ulcer. Currently,

TABLE 5.1. DIAGNOSTIC TESTS FOR PEPTIC ULCER DISEASE

TEST	DESCRIPTION
PROCEDURES FOR EXAMINING THE STOMACH AND DUODENUM	
Endoscopy (gastroscopy)	The stomach and duodenum are examined through an endoscope for ulcers and tumors. Tissue biopsy samples can be taken by means of small forceps on the endoscope. These samples can be examined for malignancy and the presence of *H. pylori* bacteria.
Radiography (upper GI series)	The stomach and duodenum—the upper gastrointestinal (GI) tract—are X-rayed for the presence of ulcers and tumors.
Computed tomography (CAT scan)	Two- or three-dimensional X-ray images of the stomach or duodenum are examined for perforations and intestinal obstructions.
Ultrasound	Sonogram images are made of the stomach and duodenum. (This test is not especially useful to peptic ulcer patients.)
BIOPSY TESTS FOR DETECTING *H. PYLORI* INFECTION	
Rapid urea (RUT)	Biopsy tissue samples are tested for the presence of urease, a byproduct of *H. pylori*. If urease is present, the patient is infected.
Culture	Bacteria from a biopsy tissue sample are cultured in a lab and examined to find out whether the tissue contains *H. pylori* bacteria.
Histologic	A biopsy tissue sample is stained with different dyes and examined under a microscope to see whether it contains *H. pylori* bacteria.
Polymerase chain reaction (PCR) assay	Samples are amplified, or copied, by means of PCR, and analyzed for *H. pylori* genes. This test offers a way to detect *H. pylori* in samples with low bacterial loads.
NONINVASIVE TESTS FOR DETECTING *H. PYLORI* INFECTION	
Urea breath	The patient's breath is tested for the presence of urease, an enzyme produced by *H. pylori*. Patients with urease in their lungs are infected.
Serological (antibody)	The patient's blood is tested for the presence of *H. pylori* antibodies. Patients with these antibodies are (or were) infected.
Other noninvasive tests	For the sake of cost and convenience, these less accurate noninvasive tests are available: stool antigen immunoassay, finger-prick blood test, and saliva test.

the most advanced procedures for detecting ulcers in the stomach and duodenum are endoscopy, radiography, computed tomography (CT), and ultrasound. Let's look at how they work and what they can reveal.

Endoscopy

An *endoscopy*, sometimes called a *gastroscopy*, is the examination of a patient's stomach and duodenum by means of an *endoscope*. This instrument is designed to permit a health practitioner to inspect the inside of the body. Endoscopes designed for peering inside the gastrointestinal tract include the gastroscope, esophagoscope, and colonoscope. An endoscope consists of a narrow, flexible tube about the width of a ball-point pen that is encased in vinyl or rubber. Fiber-optic and microchip technology in the tube light the interior of the stomach and duodenum. This technology also captures images that are recorded on a video monitor. On the monitor, circular white-gray peptic ulcers can clearly be seen against the pink mucosa of the stomach or duodenal lining. Channels in the tube provide air, suction, and water so that health practitioners—and patients, if they so choose—can get a better view of the stomach and duodenum (air inflates the stomach to make tissue more visible). By means of the suction channel and tiny forceps on the end of the instrument, practitioners can collect gastric juices and tissue samples for biopsies. These tissue samples can be examined for the presence of *H. pylori* bacteria. As part of an endoscopy, doctors can perform small-scale operations such as polyp removal, injections into bleeding sites, and tissue cauterization.

Patients must not take food for six hours or drink liquids for four hours before an endoscopy. The examination lasts ten to fifteen minutes, or a little longer if a biopsy is taken. To begin, patients' throats are sprayed with a local anesthetic to numb the area (some patients withstand the tube better than others). Apprehensive patients may be given a sedative. An endoscopy is an outpatient procedure. Typically, patients remain in the hospital after the procedure for two hours.

Endoscopy is the best way to examine the stomach and duodenum for ulcer disease. Complications from the procedure are rare, occurring in less than 1 percent of patients. Biopsies taken from the stomach or duodenum can be cultured or given a histological assessment. Examining these biopsies is the surest way to detect gastric cancer and the presence of *H. pylori* bacteria. Apart from the cost, which is considerable at roughly $1,000, there are other disadvantages of endoscopy:

- The success of the exam depends on the skill of the health practitioner. In one study, 10 percent of duodenal ulcers were not detected by endoscopy.

- Biopsies taken by endoscopy have been misdiagnosed. In a 1983 study, 4 percent of biopsies conducted by endoscopy of ulcerating gastric lesions were initially judged benign, but they turned out to be malignant when examined a second time.

However minimal, these are the risks and complications of endoscopy:

- Patients may react or be sensitive to the medication with which they are anesthetized or sedated.

- Patients may suffer from undue anxiety.

- The endoscope may injure the esophagus, stomach, or duodenum, which can cause infection.

- Vomiting can occur during the procedure and cause infection in the lungs.

Some years ago, there were reports of *H. pylori* infections being spread by contaminated endoscopes and biopsy forceps. However, the transmission of bacteria by improperly sterilized endoscopes is very rare.

Radiography

A *radiography* is a diagnostic test that provides X-ray images of the inside of the body. A radiography test that examines the esophagus, stomach, and duodenum is called an *upper gastrointestinal (GI) tract series,* or sometimes an *upper GI.* At the start of the examination, patients swallow twenty ounces of a white, chalky liquid called barium, and, in most tests, baking-soda crystals as well. Barium is a low-grade radioactive metallic solution. Its job is to make the interior surfaces of the upper GI tract more visible in X-rays. Baking-soda crystals create gas that distends the stomach and duodenum. As the bright-white, high-density barium coats the interior surfaces of the esophagus, stomach, and duodenum, a fluoroscope captures X-ray images of the upper GI tract and projects them in a video-like sequence on a monitor screen. In this way, doctors can clearly see how the GI tract is functioning. More importantly for ulcer patients, doctors can detect abnormalities on the interior surface of the stomach and duodenum. Barium fills ulcer craters so that the craters will stand out in X-rays. A tumor appears as a defect on the barium-coated surface of the stomach or duodenum.

An upper GI series exam is an outpatient procedure. It lasts one to two hours, or as long as five hours if the small intestine is examined. Patients must fast for eight hours prior to the examination. Because acid production in the stomach can lower the quality of X-ray images, patients must refrain as well from smoking, chewing gum, or taking antacids for eight hours. The barium used in the examination can cause constipation. Stools may be white for two or three days afterward.

Here are the shortcomings of radiography where ulcer patients are concerned:

- The pool of trained radiologists capable of performing upper GI tests is shrinking. Because endoscopy is now the preferred method for ulcer diagnosis, fewer radiologists are asked to perform upper GI tests. Consequently, fewer have the experience or training.

- Barium is diluted by gastric acid as it moves down the GI tract. Therefore, ulcers in the duodenum, the first portion of the small intestine, are less likely to be detected by radiography.

- Tumors and ulcer craters appear very clearly in X-rays, but superficial lesions caused by gastritis and esophagitis are harder to detect.

The risks of a radiography exam to patients are minimal:

- In rare instances, barium leaks into ulcer perforations and causes inflammation in nearby tissue.

- Barium is radioactive, although the amount of radiation to which patients are exposed is small (equivalent to the amount of background radiation you are exposed to in a sixteen-month period). Women who are pregnant or may be pregnant should not receive radiography exams.

- Very rarely, barium causes a blockage in the large intestine. For this reason, patients with a gastrointestinal obstruction should not undergo radiography.

In a *double-contrast radiography* exam, also called an air-contrast or double-contrast upper GI, patients swallow baking-soda crystals along with the barium solution. The crystals produce gas. In effect, this gas inflates the stomach and duodenum so that more surface area can be coated with barium and photographed by X-ray. Single-contrast radiography examinations in which patients don't take crystals along with barium are considered obsolete for the diagnosis of peptic ulcer disease. Barium taken by itself for a radiography test is called a single-contrast barium meal. Barium taken with baking-soda crystals is called a double-contrast barium meal.

Endoscopy vs. Radiology

For ulcer patients, an endoscopy is superior to radiography. Ulcers show up more clearly in an endoscopy, and, of course, doctors cannot take biopsy tissue samples by radiography as they can by endoscopy. However, some patients can't tolerate the discomfort of the endoscope in their throats and stomachs. For those patients, radiography may be the necessary diagnostic choice. A radiography examination costs three to four times less than an endoscopy, and endoscopies are not available in some hospitals. Numerous studies have compared the accuracy of radiography exams and endoscopies for ulcer diagnosis. In studies in which the examiners were well trained, the exams were considered of equal value for detecting ulcers as long as double-contrast radiography was used. The risks posed by endoscopy, however slight, are higher than those posed by radiography.

Computed Tomography (CT)

Computed tomography (CT), also known as a CAT (computerized axial tomography) scan, is a diagnostic technique in which X-rays of a person's body are taken simultaneously at different angles. The X-rays are assembled by computer software into two- or three-dimensional images. The medical community uses this technology widely. In 1979, Geoffrey Hounsfield and Allan Commack received the Nobel Prize in Medicine for inventing computed tomography.

During a CAT scan, patients lie in what amounts to a large X-ray tube. X-ray beams are shot through the patient's body and measured on the opposite side. A weak beam indicates bone, cartilage, or other dense tissue; a strong beam indicates soft tissue such as that found in the lungs. A computer processes these measurements and compiles them into a picture of the relative density of the tissue being examined. In this way, pictures of the interior parts of the body are formed. Most ulcer patients undergoing a CAT scan are fed a barium meal to illuminate the boundaries of the gastrointestinal tract. CAT scans are useful for detecting ulcer perforations and intestinal obstructions. They have no value for examining inflammatory gastric diseases.

Ultrasound

Ultrasound, also called *sonography* and *ultrasound scanning,* is a method of obtaining images called sonograms of the body's internal organs. Before the exam, a gel or lotion is spread over the abdomen. Then a device called a transducer is pressed against the stomach. The transducer emits inaudible, high-frequency sound waves. It also records these sounds as they echo from body tissue. Information about the pitch and strength of the reflected sound waves is sent to a computer. The computer constructs a real-time picture of the body's internal organs from reflected sound waves. The pictures are recorded on videotape or digital computer files.

Ultrasound is safe. Because it doesn't involve the use of radiation or damage body tissue, it is commonly used to monitor the development of fetuses in pregnant women. It permits doctors and patients to instantly see and examine body organs. Because images are captured in real-time, they show movement of the internal organs and tissues. This technology is not especially useful for peptic ulcer patients, because ulcers don't show very well on a sonogram. Ultrasound is only useful for detecting gallstones, tumors of the esophagus, and stomach tumors. However, ultrasound technology is improving. Doctors hope and expect that the coming years will see improvements in ultrasound that will make it a viable diagnostic technique for peptic ulcer disease. The procedure is non-invasive and it costs less than endoscopy or radiology.

BIOPSY TESTS FOR DETECTING *H. PYLORI* INFECTION

A *biopsy* is a piece of tissue that has been removed from a living body for the purpose of making a medical diagnosis. After a tissue biopsy has been obtained, usually by endoscopy, doctors can test it in various ways to see if it contains *Helicobacter pylori* (*H. pylori*) bacteria. As Chapter 2 explains, the *H. pylori* bacterium is a primary cause of peptic ulcer disease. Biopsy tests for detecting *H. pylori* bacteria include the culture test, histologic assessment, polymerase chain reaction (PCR) analysis, and rapid urea test (RUT).

Rapid Urea Test (RUT)

In a rapid urea test (RUT), a tissue sample obtained by endoscopy is incubated in agar gel containing urea and a pH-sensitive indicator. If *H. pylori* bacteria are present, the bacteria's urease enzymes react to the urea and change the color of the gel. Test results can be obtained in one day.

This test is considered 90 percent accurate, although accuracy rates are lower if the patient has recently taken bismuth or antibiotics. Larger biopsy sizes and longer incubation periods yield more accurate results. Biopsies obtained from patients with bleeding ulcers may produce false-negative results. Researchers believe this is due to excess blood in the samples. Biopsy tissue from patients with bleeding ulcers is often given a histologic assessment to confirm the results of the rapid urea test.

Several commercial rapid urea tests are available, the most popular being the CLO test (Campylobacter-Like Organism test). This test was developed by Barry Marshall, the co-discoverer of *H. pylori*. Why the odd name? Because when the test was devised in 1988, *Helicobacter pylori* was thought to belong to the genus *Campylobacter,* and the bacterium was called *Campylobacter pylori.*

Histologic Assessment

Histology is the study of cells under a microscope. In a histologic assessment, a tissue biopsy is stained with various dyes to make the cells' shape, structure, color, and growth patterns stand out. Then the cells are studied under a microscope. In the case of *H. pylori* histologic assessments, lab technicians look for the tell-tale structures and growth patterns of *H. pylori* bacteria. Histologic assessment is considered the "gold standard" of *H. pylori* diagnoses. The accuracy of other tests is measured against histologic evaluations. However, studies have shown that staining methods influence the accuracy of detections. In a study conducted in Cambridge, England, of labs using hematoxylin and eosin staining, the overall detection rate in positive *H. pylori* samples was only 66 percent. Results of histologic assessments take at least two days to complete. This is the most expensive *H. pylori*-detection test. Biopsy tissue judged negative by rapid urease testing is sometimes given a histologic assessment to be certain that *H. pylori* is not present in the tissue.

Culture Test

In a culture test, the tissue biopsy is sent to a lab, where bacteria from the tissue are cultured and studied. To culture bacteria, a tissue sample is placed on an agar plate and allowed to incubate for three to five days. During this time, the bacteria multiply and form colonies. To identify the bacteria, researchers examine their shape, size, and gram-stain color under a microscope.

The advantage of the culture testing method is that physicians can determine which strains of the *H. pylori* bacteria they are dealing with. They can then choose an antibiotic known to eradicate the particular *H. pylori* strain. Bacterial cultures are valuable because researchers can store the bacteria for further study. The disadvantages of this testing method are many. Results of the test take several days to obtain. The test is expensive and prone to error. With a sensitivity rate of 77 to 95 percent, the test is not considered highly accurate.

Polymerase Chain Reaction (PCR) Test

A *polymerase chain reaction* (PCR) is a biochemical procedure through which a DNA segment from a mixture of DNA chains can be quickly amplified or cloned to make millions of duplicate copies. In terms of peptic ulcer disease, PCR can be useful in detecting the presence of *H. pylori* bacteria when doctors have only very small samples with which to work.

PCR is quite new—it was invented in the mid-1980s by Dr. Kary Mullis, the winner of the 1993 Nobel Prize in chemistry. Its application in identifying *H. pylori* bacteria in samples has not been fully refined or standardized, but early studies are promising. In 2003, researchers at the Kaohsiung Medical University Hospital in Kaohsiung, Taiwan undertook an experiment involving PCR and gastric juice samples. The bacterial load in gastric juice is very low—far lower than the bacterial load in a tissue biopsy. Nevertheless, the Taiwanese scientists wanted to see if they could use the PCR technique to create copies of microbial DNA in gastric juice and use it for identification purposes.

In the experiment, forty-eight subjects with dyspepsia were given standard *H. pylori* detection tests, including rapid urease tests, urea breath tests, tissue culture tests, and histologic assessments. Then gastric juice samples were taken from the subjects and analyzed by polymerase chain reaction for the presence of *H. pylori*. All tests revealed that thirty-four of the forty-eight subjects were infected by *H. pylori*. PCR analyses found *H. pylori* in thirty-two of the thirty-four subjects for a respectable sensitivity rating of 94 percent. (Sensitivity rating is a measure of how efficient a test is.) PCR detection rates, the scientists reported, were comparable to those of rapid urease and urea breath tests, and superior to those of tissue culture and histologic assessments.

In the study, gastric juice samples from patients were obtained by means of the string test. In this test, fasting patients swallow a very lightweight nylon string coiled in a gelatin capsule. The end of the string is taped to the subject's cheek so it can't be swallowed as the string uncoils. After an hour or more, the string is retrieved, and gastric juice on the string is analyzed. Although string tests do not yield nearly as much bacteria as endoscopies, they cost less and do not cause as much discomfort for patients.

The PCR technique holds promise as a way of detecting *H. pylori* infections from gastric juice obtained by the string test. The problem with the PCR technique, however, is that *H. pylori* strains are genetically diverse. This can make the genetic fingerprinting of *H. pylori* by polymerase chain reaction difficult. More studies are needed in this area of testing.

NONINVASIVE TESTS FOR DETECTING *H. PYLORI* INFECTION

A noninvasive test does not require an apparatus that enters the body or breaks the skin. Generally speaking, these tests do not cost as much as invasive tests or submit patients to as much discomfort. Typically, however, they are not as accurate as invasive tests. Noninvasive tests for detecting *H. pylori* include the urea breath test, serological (antibody) tests, and various tests performed on stool, saliva, and whole blood that is obtained by pricking the skin. Let's examine these tests.

Urea Breath Test

In order to survive in the stomach's harsh acidic environment, *H. pylori* emit an enzyme called urease. This enzyme breaks down urea, a substance found in saliva and the stomach's gastric juices, to create ammonia and carbon dioxide, and these chemicals, in turn, neutralize stomach acid and help *H. pylori* survive. The urea breath test detects whether urea, and therefore *H. pylori*, is present in the patient's stomach. Tests are mailed to a laboratory for analysis and the results are usually available in two days. The test is 80 to 90 percent accurate and it costs $200 to $300.

For the test, the patient swallows a capsule that contains Carbon-13 or Carbon-14 urea. If *H. pylori* are present in the stomach, the bacteria see the urea coming, emit the urease enzyme, and break down the urea into carbon dioxide. This carbon dioxide is absorbed through the stomach and into the bloodstream. From there, it is excreted from the lungs and exhaled in the patient's breath for a positive test result. If *H. pylori* are not present in the stomach, the urea does not break down. Instead of being absorbed into the stomach, it passes out of the body in the urine and does not register in the breath test. Breath samples are taken ten to twenty minutes after the urea capsule is swallowed.

Two types of carbon isotope, Carbon-13 (^{13}C) and Carbon-14 (^{14}C), can be administered for the test. The ^{14}C isotope is radioactive, so it is not used on children or pregnant women, although the level of radiation in the isotope is equivalent to the level of radiation in a chest X-ray.

For the test to be reliable, patients must not have taken bismuth (Pepto-Bismol) or antibiotics for four weeks. They must not have taken proton pump inhibitors (omeprazole, lansoprazole, panoprazole, or others) for two weeks.

Serological

A serological test, better known as a blood test, checks for the presence of anti-*H. pylori* IgG (immunoglobulin G) antibodies in blood samples. Your body produces antibodies to fight bacterial infections, *H. pylori* included. If you have been exposed to *H. pylori*, your blood carries anti-*H. pylori* IgG antibodies to fight this particular invader.

Commercial serological test kits for detecting anti-*H. pylori* antibodies are called ELISA (enzyme-linked immunosorbent assay) tests. Several companies manufacture ELISA test kits. Test results are thought to be 90 percent accurate, although a recent analysis of eleven commercial test kits by Loy et al. reduced the accuracy rate to 85 percent or lower. Because the accuracy rate of ELISA tests are debated in the medical community, patients with peptic ulcer disease who are likely to be infected by *H. pylori* are often given a second test if their ELISA test results are negative. Unlike the urea breath test, taking antibiotics, bismuth, or proton pump inhibitors does not invalidate the results of a serological test.

Anti-*H. pylori* antibodies remain in the blood for a year or more after *H. pylori* bacteria have been eradicated. Antibody tests really only show whether you were infected during the previous two years. They don't reveal whether you are currently infected by *H. pylori*.

Other Noninvasive Tests

Doctors may also use the following *H. pylori*-detection tests:

- **Stool antigen immunoassay.** An antigen is any substance that provokes the immune system to respond. The stool antigen test detects substances that provoke the immune system to respond to an invasion by *H. pylori*. If these antigens are found in the stool, the test is positive and the patient has been infected. Results can be obtained in about three hours.

- **Finger-prick blood test.** This test detects anti-*H. pylori* antibodies in whole blood, not blood serum. Several kits have been approved by the FDA. The tests cost about $25. Results are available in five to fifteen minutes.

- **Saliva test.** Saliva samples are tested for anti-*H. pylori* antibodies by enzyme-linked immunosorbent assay (ELISA). Tests are believed to be 80 percent accurate.

These noninvasive tests are not as accurate as serological or urea breath tests, but, in light of cost and convenience, or simply to get a preliminary diagnosis, doctors may consider using them.

CONCLUSION

Every ulcer has the potential to hemorrhage. If the ulcer crater lies on an important artery, the potential danger of massive bleeding is higher. For these reasons, it is very important to consult a physician if you have three or more of the following five common ulcer symptoms: abdominal pain, meal-related pain, dyspepsia, trouble sleeping because of stomach pain that occurs at night, and, of course, bloody vomit or bloody stools.

The good news for ulcer sufferers is that modern diagnostic techniques have made it possible for doctors to diagnose an ulcer with near 100-percent certainty. Doctors and their patients can choose between noninvasive tests, such as the urea breath test or finger-prick blood test, or they can opt for invasive yet more thorough tests, such as an endoscopy or a radiological exam.

In the next chapter, I explain what happens when a diagnosis is positive, and present standard conventional drug treatments for peptic ulcer disease.

6

Conventional
Ulcer Treatments

Now that we have examined what ulcers are, what causes
them, and how to know if we have them, let's look at how
modern medicine treats this condition. In this chapter, I will
explain how doctors treat peptic ulcer disease with over-the-counter (OTC) remedies, prescription drugs, and surgical techniques.
The last thirty years have witnessed a number of innovations for
treating peptic ulcer disease with drugs. Prior to 1970, doctors had
to rely on antacids and bismuth to relieve most peptic ulcer pain.
Now, they can choose from an array of powerful drugs and drug
combinations that relieve pain, increase the stomach's defenses,
eradicate *H. pylori* bacteria, and, last but not least, heal ulcers.
However, with that said, it is important to point out that many of
these medications also come with potential side effects, which I
will discuss as well.

All OTC remedies and prescription drugs fall into three
categories:

- Medications that neutralize gastric acid or inhibit the production of gastric acid. These drugs include antacids, H_2-blocking
  drugs (H_2 receptor antagonists), and proton pump inhibitors
  (PPIs).

- Medications and natural supplements that bolster the stomach's
  mucosal defenses against harm from gastric acid. These medications include sucralfate, prostaglandin analogs, and bismuth.
  Zinc-Carnosine, a natural supplement, also improves the stom-

ach's mucosal defenses and is well worth considering as a way to heal your ulcer.

- Antibiotics that eradicate *H. pylori* bacteria in the stomach and duodenum. As explained in Chapter 2, *H. pylori* may be responsible for as many as 75 percent of stomach ulcers and 90 percent of duodenal ulcers.

In this chapter, I will detail the medications and prescription drugs that fall in these categories. I will explore the benefits of Zinc-Carnosine in Chapter 8.

ANTACIDS

Antacids are designed to temporarily relieve the overt symptoms of gastric distress. They are not the best treatment for peptic ulcer disease—far from it. Antacids do not eradicate *H. pylori* bacteria. They do not offer the same long-lasting relief from stomach pain. Because they have to be taken many times a day, they do not offer the same convenience of use as H_2-blocking drugs or proton pump inhibitors. However, antacid tablets, powders, and liquids can be purchased without a prescription. They are available in every drugstore and supermarket in the United States.

A roll of antacid tablets costs little more than a roll of Lifesavers and, indeed, many of them are formulated to taste just like a sweet. It is, therefore, no wonder that a good number of people gobble antacid tablets like candy. Although sales of over-the-counter antacid tablets have been dropping due to competition from H_2 blockers and increasing awareness among consumers as to what antacids really do, antacids remain one of the bestselling over-the-counter medications in the United States. Annual sales estimates range from $2 to $3 billion.

How Antacids Work

Antacids work by neutralizing hydrochloric acid (HCl), the acid produced in the stomach to break down food and kill bacteria and other germs. HCl is extremely caustic (masons use a substance with a similar chemical composition called muriatic acid to clean mortar from bricks). Irritation to the stomach lining by HCl is responsible for most abdominal pain. Besides neutralizing HCl, some antacids produce carbon dioxide gas. When this gas reaches a certain volume, you belch. Belching relieves the pressure and pain caused by bloating in the stomach. Liquid antacids work faster than tablets because they dissolve faster in the stomach. An antacid can relieve stomach pain for two hours, at the most.

Food exits the stomach about an hour after eating. The best time to take an antacid tablet is one hour after a meal, when the stomach has emptied and the HCl content of the stomach is higher in the absence of food. The production of HCl is highest at night, between midnight and about three o'clock. Sleepwalking patients with stomach ulcers have the advantage of being able to take an antacid for the relief of pain without waking up, but all others must arise from sleep, usually on account of sharp abdominal pains, to take an antacid tablet.

Originally, it was thought that antacids provide relief solely by defusing HCl, but studies done in the early 1990s suggest that the tablets may also have a protective effect on the cells of the stomach lining. Antacids may provoke the release of prostaglandins, the hormone-like substances that regulate pain messaging and the stomach's mucosal defenses (prostaglandins are explained in Chapter 3). In addition, antacids may stimulate the stomach's secretion of mucus and bicarbonates. However, follow-up studies to those made in the early 1990s have not been undertaken, and, it appears that the stomach-protecting benefits of taking antacid tablets may result from aluminum hydroxide in the tablets—a substance known to cause harmful side effects.

Components of Antacid Medications

Not all antacids are the same. They all have different formulas usually containing a combination of different ingredients. These ingredients function differently to relieve various symptoms. As is the case with all types of self-medication, it is important to know what the individual ingredients do and do not do. It is also equally vital that you are aware of any potential downsides, or side effects, of the medicine.

Calcium Carbonate (Chalk)

Calcium carbonate—the chief mineral found in chalk—is the most effective antacid for neutralizing HCl, but the long-term consequences of taking antacids with calcium are disconcerting. One-third of the calcium in antacids bypasses the stomach, is absorbed in the small intestine, and enters the blood. Too much calcium in the blood can overwhelm the kidneys, cause kidney stones, or cause a disease called hypercalcemia, when the amount of calcium in the blood overwhelms the kidneys' ability to regulate calcium excretion. Especially if you enjoy eating dairy products, which contain calcium, don't take more than three grams of calcium-containing antacids per day. Calcium sometimes causes acid rebound, when parietal cells in the stomach, stimulated by calcium, actually increase their production of HCl after a period of two to three hours. Brand names of antacids containing calcium include Tums and Titralac.

Sodium Bicarbonate (Baking Soda)

Antacids in this category are effervescent. They react with HCl to produce copious amounts of carbon dioxide, and, consequently, belching. Sodium, a component of salt, is easily absorbed by the small intestine. Taking sodium-bicarbonate antacids is harmful to people with high blood pressure and heart disease who are trying to lower their salt intake. Of all the antacids, those containing sodium bicarbonate do the least to neutralize HCl. Brand names of such antacids include Alka-Seltzer and Bromo-Seltzer.

Magnesium Hydroxide and Aluminum Hydroxide

These two ingredients are often used in combination. Magnesium is a potent antacid, but, unfortunately, it also causes diarrhea in 25 percent of people. To compensate, manufacturers include aluminum hydroxide, which causes constipation, in their products. Aluminum has been implicated in Alzheimer's disease. It robs the body of phosphate and can cause osteoporosis. Antacids containing aluminum hydroxide also interfere with pepsin in the stomach. This enzyme breaks down dietary protein into peptides and amino acids so protein can be absorbed. People who take antacids habitually do not get as much protein—which is necessary for building muscle tissue and increasing stamina—from their diet. Brand names of such antacids include Maalox and Mylanta.

So, the next time you go shopping for antacid tablets in your drugstore or supermarket, make sure to take note of the ingredients listed on the labels. You now know why.

Side Effects of Long-Term Antacid Use

Taking the occasional antacid tablet does no harm, but their habitual use can have harmful consequences. Besides the side effects described previously, let's look at other long-term side effects of taking antacids.

Like all drugs that hinder hydrochloric acid (HCl) in the stomach, antacids reduce the stomach's natural defenses. Decreased acidity in the stomach permits more bacteria and germs to survive. In a study done with a simulated digestive tract and antacids, a poisonous bacterium found in oysters called *Vibrio vulnificus* that is normally killed by HCl, was able to survive.

Antacids can also affect the release-timing of medications. Most medications are designed to break down and be absorbed in the small intestine; but, decreases in stomach acidity can cause a medication to enter the small intestine before it is sufficiently dissolved. The medication may break down later than it is supposed to and be rendered inactive. If you are taking a medication, consider an alternative to antacids for heartburn relief.

Just as insidious, by masking the symptoms of your problem, you allow it time to get worse. I understand that we live in a society that makes it all too easy to use antacids to treat a chronic condition, but remember this: You would not put a Band-Aid on a cut that requires stitches and then forget about it. You would seek out medical attention. The same holds true for the habitual use of antacids.

H_2-BLOCKING DRUGS (H_2 RECEPTOR ANTAGONISTS)

H_2-blocking drugs, also known as H_2 receptor antagonists, work by obstructing a histamine (H) cell receptor called histamine$_2$ (H_2). While this may sound a bit technical, in essence the drugs' actions

Antacids as Calcium Supplements

Over the last decade, a tremendous amount of media attention has focused on the problem of osteoporosis—and rightfully so. In a bid to increase sales, however, makers of antacids that contain calcium carbonate have been marketing their products to elderly people with osteoporosis and others at risk for bone loss. Calcium is necessary for strong bones and teeth. According to the National Academy of Sciences Institute of Medicine, adults need about 1,000 milligrams of calcium each day. The World Health Organization recommends 800 milligrams daily. Some antacid manufacturers have touted their products as a calcium supplement as well as an antacid.

But, in reviewing the literature, one of the problems of using antacids as a source of calcium has to do with vitamin D. Studies show that calcium is absorbed more thoroughly when it is accompanied by vitamin D. A good absorbable calcium supplement, therefore, should also contain vitamin D, but calcium-carbonate antacids, of course, do not contain this vital ingredient.

Moreover, the same problems that occur when taking an antacid for a long period of time apply as well when the antacid is also a calcium supplement. Antacids interfere with normal stomach metabolism. They allow bacteria that would normally die to survive in the stomach. They hide long-term health problems and sometimes prevent medicines from being properly absorbed. As a result, the long-term consequences of taking an antacid as a calcium supplement can be harmful.

Putting aside for a moment the long-term health risks of taking calcium-carbonate antacids, it is my belief that a medication specifically designed for treating heartburn should not be treated as a calcium supplement unless it has been proven to be so. If you are worried about osteoporosis or a lack of calcium in your diet, learn as much as you can about the problem and what you can do about it from reliable sources.

simply slow down the production of hydrochloric acid in the stomach. Because the ulcers are not being irritated by stomach acid, they have a better chance of healing. Meanwhile, ulcer pain subsides.

In the 1970s, before *H. pylori* bacteria were considered a culprit, H_2 blockers were the drugs of choice for treating most peptic ulcer disease. Today, H_2 blockers still remain popular with peptic ulcer patients and those who suffer from heartburn and gastroesophageal reflux disease (GERD). These drugs are relatively inexpensive and relatively safe. The biggest plus is that patients don't have to interrupt their sleep to take a tablet or pill because H_2 blockers suppress acid production for twenty-four hours.

H_2 blockers were initially only available as prescription drugs, but they are now sold over-the-counter. Doctors sometimes recommend them for relieving ulcer pain during a treatment for an *H. pylori* infection. Although the drugs are not helpful against stomach ulcers, they can cure duodenal ulcers in six to eight weeks. However, this is possible only if they are taken at four times the dosage recommended on the product label—not something any doctor would recommend. The following H_2 blockers have been approved by the Federal Drug Administration: cimetidine (Tagamet), famotidine (Pepsid), nizatidine (Axid), and ranitidine (Zantac).

How H_2-Blocking Drugs Work

Think of a cell receptor as a kind of window through which cells communicate with one another. Cells on the papillae (the little bumps) of your tongue, for example, contain many different receptors for registering many different tastes—sweet, sour, and so on. When a sugar molecule binds to a sugar cell receptor on your tongue, your body understands that the food in your mouth is sweet and worth swallowing. A reaction ensues. Your salivary glands secrete saliva and your stomach secretes gastric acid for the purpose of digestion. H_2-blocking drugs obstruct histamine$_2$ (H_2) cell receptors in the cells lining the stomach wall. These cells are involved in the production of hydrochloric (HCl) acid. By blocking H_2 cell receptors, the drugs inhibit the production of HCl and relieve ulcer pain. H_2-blocking drugs are, in fact, antihistamines, except that they affect the histamine reaction in the stomach that is involved in HCl production, not the histamine reaction in the nose and throat.

What Are Antihistamines?

In 1942, my father, Dr. Bernard Halpern, conducted experiments with antihistamines that would prove useful for the invention of H_2-blocking drugs. My father developed the first synthetic antihistamine. His goal was to block histamine receptors so that the histamine portion of the allergic reaction would not cause hives, runny noses, itching, and constricted breathing. Today, antihistamines—anti-H_1 receptors—such as diphenhydramine (Benadryl) and dimenhydrinate (Dramamine) are sold over-the-counter for the treatment of hay fever, hives, and skin rashes. Doctors also prescribe powerful antihistamines for more serious illnesses, such as asthma.

Histamine plays a role in allergic reactions. When someone encounters an allergen for the first time—for example, pollen, cat fur, dust mites, or a mold—the person's B-cells produce large numbers of antibodies of the type that are designed to counteract the allergen. The antibodies attach themselves to cells in the nose, tongue, skin, and gastrointestinal tract. Next time the person is exposed to the allergen, the antibodies help to release histamine. The histamine binds to histamine cell receptors in body tissue, and the result is an allergic reaction. Histamine dilates the blood vessels. It causes the glands in the nose and respiratory passages to produce mucus. An allergic reaction—a histamine response—can cause sneezing, itching, watery eyes, and hives. In extreme cases, it can constrict breathing and cause an asthma attack.

For his experiments with antihistamines, my father used guinea pigs that were allergic to egg whites. Using an aerosol nebulizer, he had the guinea pigs inhale egg whites to induce an allergic reaction. The animals

Side Effects of H_2 Blockers

An enormous number of studies have been done on H_2 blockers, and all agree that the drugs are safe if they are taken at the recommended dosage. In men, cimetidine (Tagamet) effects the hypothalamus, the connection center between the brain and hormone production. H_2 blockers may cause a loss of sex drive, gynecomastia (the development of breasts), and impotence, but these side developed very severe asthma and went into shock due to the release of histamine in their bodies. Then, my father injected the guinea pigs with an antihistamine to halt the allergic reaction. The guinea pigs started breathing normally. Instead of remaining in shock, they exhibited normal behavior. All went well for the guinea pigs, but only for a short time, because soon they took a turn for the worse and died of acute bleeding stomach ulcers.

The antihistamine drug, although it blocked the histamine response in the guinea pig's nose, throat, and lungs, failed to block it in the stomach. The stomach did not respond like the other parts of the body did to the effects of the antihistamine. My father concluded that the guinea pigs died because the histamine-response mechanism in the nose, throat, and lungs is somehow different from the histamine-response mechanism in the stomach.

Thanks in part to work begun by my father, and thanks especially to J.W. Black, who received the 1988 Nobel Prize in Medicine for his work on beta-blockers and H_2 receptor antagonists, scientists were able to distinguish between two types of histamine (H) cell receptors, H_1 and H_2. The H_1 receptors on cells in the nose, throat, and lungs are involved in allergic reactions. Antihistamine drugs such as diphenhydramine and dimenhydrinate block H_1 cell receptors, and, in so doing, they prevent the histamine reactions that cause hay fever and constricted breathing. H_2 receptors in the parietal cells of the stomach are involved in the secretion of hydrochloric acid. H_2 receptor antagonists such as cimetidine and ranitidine block H_2 receptors in the stomach's parietal cells, and, in so doing, they hinder the production of hydrochloric acid and relieve ulcer pain.

effects are rare and are reversed when the drug is discontinued or patients take a different H_2 blocker. Ranitidine (Zantac) has been known to mask the symptoms of stomach cancer and delay stomach cancer diagnoses. For that reason, the drug is only prescribed when stomach cancer has been ruled out.

Also of concern is the fact that H_2 blockers affect the absorption of other drugs. Food doesn't affect the absorption rate of H_2 blockers, but sucralfate decreases the absorption rate by as much as thirty percent. Some medications pass into the intestines before they are properly absorbed; others are rendered more potent by the absence of stomach acid. If you are taking another medication as well as an H_2 blocker, alert your doctor. Your doctor may recommend a different anti-acid medication.

Finally, the real danger in taking H_2 blockers is that many people do not take the recommended dose or do not take the drugs under the supervision of a doctor. Because H_2 blockers are sold over-the-counter, people are more likely to take the drugs at higher doses. Someone with ulcer pain quickly learns that the recommended dose of two 200 mg tablets twice a day doesn't do the job, so that person doubles the dose and takes 400 mg twice a day. This can have long-term health consequences, because H_2 blockers interfere with the metabolism of the stomach. Protein and vitamin B_{12} in the diet, for example, are not absorbed properly because there isn't enough acid in the stomach to break down and absorb protein and vitamin B_{12}. Toxins and bacteria that would normally be killed by stomach acid are allowed to survive. If you are taking over-the-counter H_2 blockers, I strongly recommend seeing a physician every six months. He or she can determine whether your consumption of these drugs is doing long-term damage.

PROTON PUMP INHIBITORS (PPIS)

By far the best therapy for suppressing hydrochloric acid in the stomach is the proton pump inhibitor (PPI), also called the acid pump inhibitor. These drugs work by decreasing the production of hydrochloric acid in the stomach, relieving ulcer pain, and lessening the irritation that acid causes for ulcer sores. Since the FDA approved the first proton pump inhibitor, omeprazole (Prilosec), in 1989, these drugs have replaced H_2 blockers as the preferred means of anti-acid therapy. Besides peptic ulcers, PPIs are used to treat heartburn, gastroesophageal reflux disease (GERD), and Zollinger-Ellison syndrome. The drugs are also used in combination with antibiotics to treat *H. pylori* infections. Proton pump inhibitors are sometimes called the "zole" drugs because their names all end in *zole:* esomeprazole (Nexium), lansoprazole (Prevacid), omeprazole

(Prilosec, Losec), pantoprazole (Protonix), and rabeprazole (Aciphex). The only disadvantage of this drug compared to other anti-acid drugs is the cost, which is high. Because of its cost, some patients opt for other treatments.

How PPIs Works

On the lining of the stomach are millions of parietal cells that produce hydrochloric acid. In the final step of acid production, an enzyme on the parietal cell—the proton pump—releases acid through the cell membrane into the stomach. Proton pump inhibitors target this enzyme and inactivate it. As a result, parietal cells produce less hydrochloric acid or no acid at all, and the patient feels less stomach pain. The enzyme in parietal cells responsible for releasing acid was named the "proton pump" because its biochemical name—hydrogen-potassium adenosine triphosphatase (H +, K + -ATPase)—is a mouthful in anybody's language.

PPIs are long lasting. After the drug lands in the parietal cell's secretory canal, it remains there; it is "trapped" in the cell and can't go back across the cell membrane. In time, the drug accumulates in parietal cells, which accounts for the drug's long-lastingness. Daily doses taken for three to five days have a cumulative effect so that the secretion of basic acid in the stomach is inhibited by nearly 100 percent after a week. Patients need only to take the drug once a day because it is so enduring. The effect of a single dose can remain for four days.

Therapy by proton pump inhibitors can cure an ulcer in two to four weeks. Patients usually take the drugs for one to two months at a stretch. Because the half-life of a proton pump inhibitor is eighteen hours, the secretion of hydrochloric acid by parietal cells returns to normal two to five days after the drug is discontinued.

Side Effects of PPIs

The side effects of taking proton pump inhibitors include headaches, abdominal pain, diarrhea, constipation, and flatulence. Although these side effects appear in one in twenty patients, most patients who experience side effects do so willingly in exchange for the relief from stomach pain that PPIs afford. Hydrochloric acid in the stomach kills bacteria and other germs. Of more concern to doctors than the side effects just listed are the long-term consequences of low acidity in the stomach:

- In patients who take PPIs for many months, bacteria, parasites, and germs, including *H. pylori*, may survive or colonize in the gastrointestinal tract. Bacterial microbes are responsible for the abdominal pain, diarrhea, and flatulence that sometimes accompany the use of PPIs.

- Stomach acid is necessary for the absorption of some nutrients, especially proteins and vitamin B_{12}. People who take PPIs for long periods of time may be deprived of the necessary amounts of these nutrients.

- Some drugs—most notably ketoconazole (for fungal infections), ampicillin (an antibiotic), and digoxin (for heart disease)—rely on stomach acid to be absorbed properly. Patients do not get sufficient doses of these drugs if they take them along with PPIs.

- PPIs stimulate the growth of enterochromaffin-like (ECL) cells in the stomach. In one study, rats fed omeprazole for two years developed an abnormal growth of ECL cells, and some developed gastric carcinoid tumors. Fortunately, there are no reports of humans getting these tumors.

The good news is that studies done thus far on the long-term effects of taking PPIs have given the drugs a passing grade. But these drugs are new. The prolonged suppression of acid may open the door to health complications. The next decade will reveal how safe or unsafe proton pump inhibitors really are.

PROSTAGLANDIN ANALOGS

As I explained in Chapter 3, non-steroidal anti-inflammatory drugs (NSAIDs) work by affecting hormone-like substances in the body called prostaglandins. NSAIDs relieve pain and decrease swelling by halting prostaglandin production in body tissue. However, this lack of prostaglandins has an untoward effect on the stomach. Prostaglandins are necessary for building the stomach's defensive mucosal layer. Halting their production in the stomach weakens the stomach's mucosal defenses. It exposes the stomach and duodenum to caustic gastric acid and increases the chances of getting an ulcer. The use of NSAIDs is to blame for roughly 30 percent of stomach ulcers and 10 percent of duodenal ulcers, and these numbers are rising.

How Prostaglandin Analogs Work

The idea behind prostaglandin analogs is to permit patients to take NSAIDs without the risk of getting an ulcer. Synthetic prostaglandin analogs, it is hoped, will do in the stomach what natural prostaglandins do—help build the stomach's defensive mucosal layer. The drugs are costly and present serious risks. Only people with rheumatoid arthritis and other diseases for which they must take NSAIDs to relieve pain may be given prostaglandin analogs. For people who aren't taking NSAIDs, proton pump inhibitors or H_2 blockers are the better treatment choices. Several prostaglandin analogs are available, but only misoprostol (Cytotec) has been approved by the FDA for use in the United States. The drug is not prescribed with great frequency.

Side Effects of Prostaglandin Analogs

Misoprostol causes stomach cramps—10 to 30 percent of people who take it get severe diarrhea. Postmenopausal women may experience vaginal bleeding. Prostaglandins figure in uterus contractions, and prostaglandin analogs can cause miscarriages. The drugs are used irresponsibly to self-induce abortion. Pregnant women should not take this drug.

BISMUTH

Bismuth is found in the medicine cabinets of two-thirds of American households in the form of the patent medicine Pepto-Bismol. This medication is used to treat the general symptoms of upset stomach, diarrhea, and colitis, as well as peptic ulcers. Bismuth comes from the German *wissmuth*, which means "white mass."

With the invention of H_2 blockers in the 1970s, bismuth fell out of favor as a treatment for ulcer disease, but it made a comeback starting in 1985 when Dr. Barry Marshall, the co-discoverer of *H. pylori*, used it as a companion to antibiotics in peptic ulcer treatments. Today, bismuth is used with antibiotics in triple and quadruple drug therapies to treat ulcers caused by *H. pylori* infections. Although the action of the drug is totally different, bismuth is considered the equal of H_2 blockers in its clinical results.

How Bismuth Works

Bismuth used to be considered an antacid. It turns out, however, that the drug also works by coating ulcer craters in the stomach and acting as a barrier between ulcers and hydrochloric acid. Bismuth is also a low-grade antibacterial agent. It inhibits the growth of *H. pylori*. The drug does this by detaching *H. pylori* bacteria from the stomach's mucosal layer so the microorganisms can be killed more effectively. Bismuth may also encourage the production of prostaglandins, the hormone-like substances that stimulate mucus production in the stomach and duodenum.

Two types of bismuth formulations are used to treat peptic ulcers: colloidal bismuth subcitrate (CBS) and bismuth subsalicylate (BSS). CBS is used in Europe (under the brand name De Nol) but has not been approved by the FDA in the United States. BSS, the formulation in Pepto-Bismol, has been approved by the FDA as a treatment for peptic ulcers.

Side Effects of Bismuth

Prior to the 1960s, bismuth was considered a wonder drug for the treatment of ulcers. It was available over-the-counter and widely used. The drug was especially popular with the elderly. Medicinal bismuth, however, appears to be able to cross the blood-brain barrier. In the 1960s, toxicity caused by long-term exposure to colloidal bismuth subcitrate (CBS) caused brain damage in many people who took the drug. It was taken off the shelf and strictly regulated. If bismuth is taken for longer than a week, it must be used only under the careful supervision of a doctor. I advise against using bismuth for more than two weeks under any circumstances.

Taking Pepto-Bismol causes stools to turn dark, which is harmless, but frightens some people. The drug should not be given to children because it has been implicated in Reye's syndrome, a rare disease that can cause liver failure. As a treatment for ulcers, the drug is used chiefly in combination with antibiotics in triple- and quadruple-therapies.

ANTIBIOTIC THERAPIES

Since the discovery of the *H. pylori* bacteria in 1983, combination drug treatments that include antibiotics have become the preferred method of treating ulcer patients in whom *H. pylori* is present. The bacterium is believed to cause 75 percent of stomach ulcers and 90 percent of duodenal ulcers. To treat *H. pylori*-induced ulcers, patients take one or two different antibiotics along with one or two drugs to relieve ulcer pain, usually a proton pump inhibitor, H_2 blocker, or both. To be considered successful, treatments must have eradicated *H. pylori* four weeks after the start of therapy. In 1994, the National Institutes of Health recommended giving antibiotic treatment to all patients with ulcers who tested positive for *H. pylori* infection. Patients with NSAID-caused ulcers who do not harbor the bacteria do not receive antibiotic treatments.

How Antibiotic Therapy Works

A bacterium is a single-cell organism with a single DNA chromosome. Bacteria can divide and reproduce very quickly. In effect, an antibiotic is a selective poison. Antibiotics are designed to kill single-cell bacterial microorganisms, but not cells in the body. Antibiotics kill bacteria in different ways. Some antibiotics destroy the cell walls or membranes of bacteria; others prevent bacterial cells from synthesizing the proteins that are necessary for building the cell's structure; others impede the bacterial cell's ability to produce new DNA.

Combination Treatments

Table 6.1 on page 118 lists antibiotics that are commonly used to treat *H. pylori* infections by their drug name and brand names. As explained in Chapter 2, *H. pylori* are durable, elusive bacteria. They

TABLE 6.1. ANTIBIOTICS FOR TREATING H. PYLORI INFECTIONS

ANTIBIOTIC	BRAND NAME(S)
amoxicillin	Amoxil, Larotid, Moxlin, Polymox, Trimox, Wymox
clarithromycin	Biaxin
metronidazole	Flagyl, Noritate, Protostat
tetracycline	Achromycin, Panmycin, Robitet, Sumycin, Tetracyn

are capable of burrowing deep into the mucosal lining of the stomach, where, out of reach of gastric acid, they can thrive and grow. To increase the chances of eradicating elusive *H. pylori* bacteria, treatments usually require two weeks and entail taking two antibiotics, instead of one. This gives the antibiotics enough strength and staying power to eradicate *H. pylori*.

To relieve ulcer pain during the treatment, patients also take one or two acid-suppressing drugs along with their antibiotics. Table 6.2 on page 119 lists the most common drug combinations for treating *H. Pylori*-caused ulcers. A triple therapy of metronidazole, tetracycline, and bismuth taken for fourteen days is the standard in the United States. Success rates of double, triple, and quadruple therapies range from 65 to 90 percent. The length of treatment ranges from seven to fourteen days.

Numerous studies have been done comparing drug combinations and dosages for treating ulcers caused by *H. pylori*. Unfortunately, these studies are difficult to compare. Some studies are better than others at monitoring subjects to make sure they really take the drugs. Subjects take different dosages of the various drugs. The individual drugs and drug combinations produce different side effects. All this adds up to a great degree of uncertainty as to which drug combination, at which dose, for which time period, works best at eradicating *H. pylori* and healing ulcers.

I tend to agree with the dual-therapy regimen of taking clarithromycin along with bismuth or an anti-acid drug for seven days. This is the therapy used in Europe. Clarithromycin works fast, well, and for an extended period of time. Triple and quadruple therapies are expensive. They are an enormous inconvenience

TABLE 6.2. DRUG COMBINATION TREATMENTS FOR *H. PYLORI*-INDUCED ULCERS		
REGIMEN	ANTIBIOTIC(S)	OTHER DRUG(S)
Dual therapy	amoxicillin	PPI*
	clarithromycin	PPI*
Triple therapy	metronidazole, tetracycline	bismuth
	clarithromycin, metronidazole	PPI*
	amoxicillin, clarithromycin	PPI*
	amoxicillin, metronidazole	PPI*
	tetracycline, metronidazole	sucralfate
Quadruple therapy	metronidazole, tetracycline	bismuth, H_2 blocker
	metronidazole, amoxicillin	bismuth, H_2 blocker
	metronidazole, tetracycline	bismuth, PPI*
	metronidazole, clarithromycin	bismuth, PPI*

* Protein pump inhibitor

for patients, who sometimes must take as many as a dozen tablets per day for two weeks. Patients are more likely to comply with the dual-therapy regimen because it doesn't make as many demands on them. In studies, the success rate of triple and quadruple therapies is higher than that of dual therapies, but not especially higher. If studies factored compliancy rates into their analyses of *H. pylori* treatments, dual therapy might well come out ahead of triple and quadruple therapy.

Resistance to Antibiotics

When antibiotics were introduced in the 1940s, they were presented to the public as a kind of miracle drug. And antibiotics have performed many miracles. Death by infectious bacterial disease is one-twentieth what it was a hundred years ago. In 1900, hospitals were very dangerous places. If bacteria entered and infected a surgical incision, the patient often died.

The trouble with antibiotics, however, is that bacteria find ways to resist them. Some bacteria are very resilient. As they fight off antibiotics, they develop into new strains—strains that are resistant. For example, *Streptococcus pneumoniae,* a bacterium that causes pneumonia and meningitis, used to be treatable by penicillin, but some strains have become resistant. Now, the bacterium causes a half-million cases of pneumonia and an estimated seven to ten million ear infections in children annually. Bacterial resistance is caused by natural selection. The antibiotic kills most bacteria, but the strongest survive and hand down their survival characteristics to the next generation. It appears that some bacteria train plasmids to convey resistance to other bacterial species.

Microarray analyses of *H. pylori* have determined that three-fourths of the bacterium's genes are the same from strain to strain, but a quarter of *H. pylori* gene sequences are specific to each strain. This indicates that the *H. pylori* bacterium is genetically diverse and, therefore, capable of many permutations. One study found that *H. pylori* resistance to metronidazole is 95 percent in South Korea. Although methods of defining the resistance of the bacteria to antibiotics have not been standardized, this study and others like it suggest that resistant *H. pylori* strains are appearing on the scene.

Besides bacterial resistance, the other drawback of antibiotic treatments is the problem of re-infection. In the crowded slums of the developing world, *H. pylori* bacteria are everywhere. A person who is successfully treated for an *H. pylori* infection may be re-infected shortly afterward.

Side Effects of Antibiotics

Antibiotics that are used to treat *H. pylori* infections fall into the following categories:

- **Macrolides.** The number of allergies to these antibiotics is limited. However, they irritate the intestines and often cause diarrhea. Clarithromycin (brand name Biaxin) is in the macrolides category.

- **Flagyl.** This antibiotic interferes with the metabolism of alcohol, and people taking it should abstain from alcohol in any form (vinegar included). It is also a photosensitizer that makes the skin very susceptible to sunburn. This antibiotic is inexpensive and works very fast.

- **Tetracycline.** This antibiotic is well tolerated. However, like flagyl, it is a photosensitizer. It should not be given to pregnant women or children because it affects the growth of bones and teeth.

- **Ampicillin, amoxicillin.** These antibiotics are very well tolerated and for that reason are the standard antibiotic given to children for bacterial infections. A very limited number of people develop severe allergic reactions to these antibiotics. Anyone who takes them and experiences hives, swelling of the face, or shortness of breath should go to the hospital immediately.

When patients are given an antibiotic that they have never taken before, they should be monitored for allergic reactions.

SUCRALFATE

Sucralfate (brand names Sulcrate, Antipepsin, Carafate) is not a first-line ulcer treatment. The drug is used to treat ulcers chiefly in Japan. Except for its short-term soothing effect on stomach ulcer pain, it has become largely obsolete. Since the advent of PPIs and H_2 blockers, its prescription rate has dropped dramatically, although some doctors still favor it in triple-therapy treatments for *H. pylori*-caused ulcers, and it is sometimes prescribed if PPIs and H_2 blockers don't work.

Sucralfate must be taken on an empty stomach. Because the drug works for only six hours, patients must take it throughout the day. The pills are large and difficult to swallow (the medical literature includes the tale of an unfortunate man who got a gastric bezoar formation, an undissolved sucralfate pill, stuck in his stomach). Sucralfate impairs the absorption of some antibiotics, so it cannot be used in combination with certain antibiotics to treat *H. pylori*-induced ulcers. It has not been approved by the FDA for the treatment of ulcers.

How Sucralfate Works

Sucralfate works like a sticky paste to coat ulcerated tissue and prevent its exposure to hydrochloric acid (HCl), bile salts, pepsinogen, and other caustic substances. Some studies show that sucralfate reduces HCl production, but the drug itself does little to neutralize HCl. Another study presented sucralfate as suppressing, but not eradicating, *H. pylori* bacteria. Sucralfate may stimulate the production of prostaglandins, the hormone-like substances involved in building the stomach's protective mucosal barrier. In one study, 70 to 80 percent of patients with duodenal ulcers who took one gram of sucralfate four times daily healed after a period of four weeks; 85 to 99 percent of patients healed after eight weeks.

Side Effects of Sucralfate

Sucralfate is composed of sucrose and aluminum-hydroxide. The aluminum causes constipation in 3 percent of patients. Apart from subjects in clinical studies, it is hard to imagine anyone undergoing a long-term treatment with sucralfate, but if someone were to do that, he or she might be exposed to exorbitant amounts of aluminum. This mineral interferes with protein absorption and has been implicated in Alzheimer's disease.

If your physician has prescribed sucralfate as an ulcer treatment, make sure you ask why. With the availability of the other drugs I have described, the use of sucralfate would be highly questionable.

SURGICAL TREATMENTS FOR BLEEDING ULCERS

Except to treat perforated ulcers and acute bleeding ulcers in emergency situations, surgery has become, thankfully, an uncommon ulcer treatment. Most emergency surgeries are performed on elderly people who take NSAIDs and begin bleeding suddenly. The mortality rate from these surgeries is relatively low, from 5 to 10 percent. In many instances, doctors can perform ulcer surgery by means of an endoscope. Using this flexible, fiberoptic instrument, doctors can cauterize ulcers to coagulate blood and stop bleeding.

Doctors rarely perform the following ulcer surgeries. If all else fails, they may have to resort to these medical procedures to cure ulcer disease:

- **Antrectomy.** Surgical removal of the antrum, or lower half of the stomach. Most stomach acid is produced, and most stomach ulcers occur, in the antrum. Removing this portion of the stomach lowers acid production and leaves a smaller stomach area in which ulcers can form.

- **Vagotomy.** The severing of the vagus nerve (the major stimulus for acid production in the stomach) to halt messages from the brain to the stomach that stimulate acid secretion. A vagotomy is performed to cease acid production in the stomach.

- **Pyloroplasty.** Enlargement of the opening from the stomach into the small intestine so that the contents of the stomach can exit more easily. A pyloroplasty widens the opening of the duodenum. The procedure is usually preformed along with a vagotomy. Cutting the vagus nerve delays the emptying of the stomach and renders the stomach inert, but a pyloroplasty permits food to leave the stomach on a more regular basis.

Until the advent of H_2 blockers in the 1970s, surgery was the treatment for severe, difficult-to-treat ulcers. Ulcer patients can count themselves lucky that surgery is rarely used today to treat ulcers.

CONCLUSION

Doctors and patients have to take into consideration many different factors when choosing the right drugs to treat peptic ulcers—if they choose to go the drug treatment route. All the drugs have side effects. When taken together, the drugs affect patients in a myriad of ways. If you found the many different drug choices that I described in this chapter perplexing, you are not alone. Medical science has given us many methods of treating peptic ulcers, but it has also made matching the patient to the right treatment harder.

In the next two chapters, I look at ways to treat peptic ulcers apart from conventional drug therapy. In Chapter 7, I explore alternative treatments; in Chapter 8, I examine the health supplement Zinc-Carnosine. The treatments I describe in the next two chapters do not act as quickly as conventional drug treatments, but in some patients they heal ulcers more thoroughly—because they work by enhancing the body's natural healing mechanisms.

7

Alternative and Complementary Treatments

For most of humankind's history, traditional methods of healing were used to treat every sort of health disorder—some successfully, some not. For centuries, tribal shamans, perhaps better known as medicine men, passed down their own local healing secrets from one generation to the next. Today, these systems of traditional medicine are still the primary healthcare methods used by most of the world's population. In China, Traditional Chinese Medicine (TCM) is practiced in hospitals alongside western medicine. The Japanese use a system called Kampo, based on an older form of today's Chinese system. In India, Ayurvedic medicine is used by a majority of its population. In Germany, all medical physicians are also trained in the use of herbs. And even in England, the royal family's physician is a homeopath.

The basis for today's modern drugs is rooted in traditional medicines. By extracting the active ingredients found in many of these folk remedies, research scientists have been able to develop more potent forms of treatment. Over the past decade in the United States, there has been a resurgence of interest in these older systems of healing. Labeled "alternative medicine," many of these treatments are now practiced throughout North America. In fact, many of today's major hospitals have complementary medicine units that work hand-in-hand with conventional physicians.

As a physician with a medical degree from the University of Paris, I have been a professor of medicine in various reputable and prestigious institutions. Throughout my medical career, I have looked with an open mind to alternative options. As I review these options, in good conscience, I can only evaluate them using the conventional methods of analysis in which I was trained. Either a natural supplement, herb, or drug passes the test of placebo-controlled study under strict medical supervision—or it simply does not pass this established test.

While the previous chapter provided you with the latest conventional treatments for peptic ulcers, in this chapter I provide you with an examination of alternative remedies. As I search the Internet, I am amazed by the volume of misleading claims that many "natural" product manufacturers make. All too many times, I am afraid that the unfounded "facts" that I read on these websites are based on greed and not science. Rather than have you guess at what's right and what's hype, I have provided you with an overview of traditional alternative remedies.

Before I begin, I would like to point out one very important fact. Alternative remedies, by their very nature, work slowly. If you have any of the symptoms that I have previously described, please seek immediate medical attention to at least establish what your problem is, and its severity. You owe it to yourself and your family to take advantage of today's modern technological wonders. Once you know what your condition is, by all means find a physician trained in gastroenterology with whom you feel comfortable—and who is open to communication. With that said, let's explore the various remedies that alternative medicine now offers to sufferers of ulcers.

HERBAL AND PLANT-BASED REMEDIES

The remedies described below come from various traditional healing systems. Some remedies are common to many; some are unique to one. The important thing to understand is how effective they are. At first glance, they may seem to have no common thread. There are vegetables, common plants, herbs, spices, and teas. When we look closer, however, we see that each individual remedy results in a beneficial biochemical reaction within the body. And, just as important, these reactions bolster or rejuvenate the body's own system of defenses. The following items have also been used by various cultures for hundreds, if not thousands, of years. They first proved useful through anecdotal evidence—that is, they were shown to work over generations without the benefit of clinical trials. The good news is that modern medicine has begun to test them, and wherever possible, I have cited these studies. So as to play no favorites among this group, I have listed them in alphabetical order.

Aloe Vera

When rubbed on the skin, the clear gel from the aloe vera plant (*Aloe barbadensis*) is used to soothe and heal sunburned skin and cuts. It was used this way by the ancient Egyptians. In European folk medicine, aloe vera juice was and is used to treat ulcers and heartburn. Taken orally, aloe vera can relieve the pain of ulcers and perhaps even help prevent the problem.

How It Works

Researchers from Barts and the London School of Medicine and Dentistry ran *in vitro* tests—in test tubes—to see what effect aloe vera gel would have on gastric cells. The aloe vera caused the cells to produce prostaglandins, the hormone-like substances responsible in part for building the stomach's protective mucosal layer. (See Chapter 3 for more information on prostaglandins.)

How To Use

If you are taking aloe vera to relieve ulcer pain, take it in small doses—one teaspoon after meals and for no more than eight weeks. After this period, consult a physician to see if your ulcer has healed.

Cautions

At high doses, aloe acts as a laxative. Avoid whole-leaf aloe vera products because they contain alloin, a cathartic, or purgative, compound that irritates the digestive tract. Instead, use gels made from the pulp of the aloe vera leaf. The translucent gel does not contain alloin.

Broccoli Sprouts

At only twenty calories, a cup of raw broccoli provides 34 mg of calcium and 66 mg of vitamin C. Phytochemicals in broccoli have significant anti-cancer effects. The vegetable's beta-carotene is an excellent antioxidant and may strengthen the immune system. And the leafy green vegetable that children and United States presidents love to hate may also be useful against *H. pylori,* the bacterium that causes stomach ulcers and stomach cancer.

How It Works

In a 2002 experiment, scientists at the Johns Hopkins University School of Medicine and the French National Scientific Research Center tested a component from broccoli sprouts called sulforaphane GS. The compound was evaluated against *H. pylori* in the test tube and against stomach ulcers in laboratory rats. The results of these experiments were encouraging.

For the test-tube part of the experiment, the scientists took stomach lining cells that were infected with *H. pylori* and subjected them to sulforaphane GS. The doctors chose stomach lining cells for the experiment because *H. pylori* bacteria are capable of burrowing deep into these cells and hiding from conventional antibiotics. For their ulcer patients, many doctors prescribe powerful combinations of two or three antibiotics because they believe that only a dose that large can reach into the stomach lining cells and kill the bacteria. In the experiment, sulforaphane GS eradicated forty-eight different strains of *H. pylori,* including some strains that have proven resistant to conventional antibiotics. Best of all, sulforaphane GS succeeded in doing this in stomach lining cells—the cells that have proven most resistant to treatment by antibiotics.

In the other half of the study, laboratory rats were given a chemical known to cause stomach cancer. Rats that were pretreated with sulforaphane GS had 39 percent fewer tumors than those who did not receive the broccoli component. Jed Fahey, the Johns Hopkins researcher who conducted the experiment, said that "The levels that are effective (in test tubes) are levels that could be achieved by eating a serving or so of broccoli sprouts, based on the chemistry we know. This isn't one of those rat studies in which you need four-hundred times the maximum amount a human could handle."

That may be so, but we still don't know whether the sulforaphane GS found in broccoli sprouts is as effective against *H. pylori* as the isolated sulforaphane GS that the Johns Hopkins scientists used in their experiment. The highest concentration of sulforaphane GS is found in broccoli sprouts, but it is also found in mature broccoli, as well as other cruciferous vegetables, including cabbage, kale, and cauliflower. The sprouts contain twenty to fifty times the concentration of sulforaphane GS as mature, cooked broccoli.

How To Use

Because broccoli sprouts are so healthy, they are now available in grocery stores. (Look for them next to the alfalfa and bean sprouts.) For more information about broccoli sprouts, go to www.broccosprouts.com. This website recommends eating one ounce (about a half cup) every other day.

Cautions

In some people, the sulfur content in broccoli sprouts can cause halitosis, commonly known as bad breath. Broccoli also predisposes people to have gas. The sulfur in broccoli can also interfere with the synthesis of thyroid hormones and can cause a goiter.

Cabbage Juice

Cabbage is rich in beta-carotene, glutamine, and vitamin C. It is an antioxidant. This fibrous vegetable is good for the gastrointestinal tract. It contains calcium, magnesium, phosphorus, potassium, sodium, copper, iron, and zinc.

How It Works

In the 1950s, Dr. Garnett Cheney of the Stanford University School of Medicine championed cabbage juice as a cure for peptic ulcers. Cabbage juice, he said, contained "vitamin U" (the U is for ulcer), a never-identified compound that gave cabbage juice its healing power over ulcer disease. The world seems to have forgotten cabbage juice as an ulcer healer in spite of these rather impressive studies conducted in the 1940s and 1950s:

- One-hundred ulcer patients drank four glasses of raw cabbage juice each day. Within one week, 81 percent of patients showed no symptoms of ulcers, and X-ray examinations confirmed that their ulcers had healed. Two-thirds of patients reported feeling better after four days.

- Thirteen ulcer patients drank a fifth of a quart of raw cabbage juice five times daily. Every patient was healed after seven to ten days.

If these studies are accurate, cabbage juice may indeed work wonders for people with ulcers. So why has cabbage juice been neglected this half century? Probably because drinking a quart or more of the vile stuff each day is too much for most people to contemplate.

How To Use
According to Dr. Cheney, it is necessary to drink four cups of cabbage juice per day to cure an ulcer. Take one cup every three to four hours.

Cautions
The side effects of drinking cabbage juice are the same as those of eating broccoli sprouts. Cabbage juice can cause halitosis and gas. It can interfere with the synthesis of thyroid hormones and produce a goiter. Of course, cabbage juice is also difficult to swallow. The British humorist William Connor said of cabbage, "Compared with boiled cabbage, steamed coarse newsprint bought from bankrupt Finnish salvage dealers and heated over smoky oil stoves is an exquisite delicacy." The only cautionary advice I have for cabbage juice drinkers is to beware of the awful flavor.

Deglycyrrhizinated Licorice (DGL)
Tea made from licorice (*Glycyrrhiza glabra*) root is a folk remedy for upset stomachs and sore throats in many different cultures. Chew-

ing the root was believed to cure viral infections. In Europe, licorice tea was a folk remedy for diarrhea. Germany's Commission E recommends taking licorice along with the chamomile flower to treat peptic ulcer disease. Deglycyrrhizinated licorice, or DGL, is a supplemental form of licorice root that provides benefits without side effects.

How It Works

Although licorice's action in the stomach isn't clearly understood, some believe that licorice stimulates the secretion of mucus and thereby fortifies the stomach's defensive mucosal layer.

Most of the evidence for DGL's effectiveness on stomach ulcers is anecdotal, but a handful of old studies are still on the books. In a 1969 study, thirty-three patients with gastric ulcers were treated with a placebo or 760 mg of DGL three times a day for one month. The authors of the study reported a 78-percent reduction in ulcer crater sizes in the DGL group compared with a 34-percent reduction in the placebo group. About 44 percent of people in the DGL group were healed of their ulcers; only 6 percent were healed in the placebo group.

In a 1979 study, researchers examined feces to determine how much blood was lost from gastric erosions caused by taking aspirin by itself and taking aspirin with DGL three times a day. Blood loss was less in those subjects who took DGL with their aspirin, which indicated that taking DGL softened the blow to the stomach lining that aspirin delivered. The study also reported that the gastric mucosal damage in rats caused by taking 60 mg of aspirin orally was reduced when the rats were also given 100 to 500 mg of deglycyrrhizinated licorice as well.

How To Use

The makers of deglycyrrhizinated licorice supplements recommend taking 300 to 400 mg per day.

Cautions

Deglycyrrhizinated licorice (DGL) is licorice with the glycyrrhizin removed. DGL produces no side effects because it contains no glycyrrhizin—a compound that can cause hypertension and water retention. Deglycyrrhizinated licorice delivers the benefits of licorice without the side effects of glycyrrhizin. (Glycyrrhizin is responsible for licorice's sweet flavor. To make commercial licorice candy, manufacturers substitute anis for glycyrrhizin.)

Fermented Foods

Fermented foods such as yogurt, kefir, sauerkraut, miso, *kim-chee*, chutney, pickled relishes, and kvass are good for your health. Nearly every civilization has a culinary tradition that includes fermented foods. Fermentation is an excellent way to keep food from spoiling and enhance a food's natural flavor. In the west, the favorite fermented food is yogurt. This natural probiotic was brought to the attention of westerners in the early 1900s by a Russian biologist named Dr. Elie Metchnikoff, a Nobel Prize winner in Medicine. Dr. Metchnikoff was very much interested in longevity, and, on a trip to the Balkan Mountains to study Bulgarian tribes (people known for their longevity), he concluded that this group of people lived long because of the yogurt in their diet. Dr. Metchnikoff took yogurt samples to his laboratory in Paris, where he isolated the bacteria in yogurt and named it *Lactobacillus bulgaricus* after the Bulgarians. He then helped establish the first yogurt producers in Europe.

How It Works

Fermented foods contain friendly bacteria—*Lactobacillus acidophillus, Lactobacillus bulgaricus, Lactobacillus plantarum, Lactobacillus casei, Bifidobacterium bifidus*, and others—that acidify the gut, making it more difficult for harmful bacteria such as *H. pylori* to survive. In effect, the lactobacilli microbes in fermented foods act as a natural antibiotic, because they colonize the intestines and crowd out harmful bacterial microbes before those microbes can get a foothold. Some strains of lactobacilli appear to prevent *H. pylori* bacteria from attaching to gastric epithelial cells. Moreover, lactobacilli can tolerate the caustic acid and bile in the gastrointestinal tract.

As early as 1985, scientists discovered that *Lactobacillus acidophilus* could eradicate *H. pylori* bacteria in the test tube. Several more studies along these lines have been undertaken in the past decade and a half:

- One-hundred-twenty *H. pylori*-infected patients were given the standard triple therapy treatment (rabeprazole, clarithromycin, and amoxicillin) for seven days. Sixty of these patients also received a *Lactobacillus acidophilus* culture three times daily. The *H. pylori*-eradication rate was higher in the *Lactobacillus acidophilus* group—86.6 percent compared with 70 percent.

- In an experiment conducted in Croatia, fourteen *H. pylori*-infected patients drank a 250 ml *Lactobacillus acidophilus* milk three times daily for two months. The patients did not receive any other therapy. At the end of two months, gastroscopies revealed that six of the fourteen patients were no longer infected by *H. pylori*.

- Scientists in Tokyo conducted an experiment on two groups of mice in which one group was fed *Lactobacillus salivarius* and then both groups were orally inoculated with *H. pylori*. The lactobacilli-fed mice were not infected with *H. pylori*, but the second group was infected and subsequently acquired gastritis.

These studies clearly show that *Lactobacillus acidophilus*, like the kind found in yogurt, halts the growth of *H. pylori* as well as other harmful microbes.

How To Use

Eat fermented food at least twice a day. When you shop for yogurt, look for the seal of the National Yogurt Association and the words "contains live active cultures." Try to buy the artisanal yogurts made by small producers. Not only do these yogurts taste better, but their bacterial cultures remain alive longer than the bacterial cultures in mass-produced brands. If the manufacturer's "use by date" has expired, don't buy the yogurt, as it will not contain active bacterial cultures.

Cautions

There are no side effects from eating fermented foods if you consume them about twice daily. I must mention again the potential problem with the commercially prepared yogurts sold in supermarkets. It is much better to get traditionally prepared fermented yogurts, which will actually contain the beneficial living organisms.

Fiber

Fiber, also known as roughage, is the indigestible remnants of plant cells in food. Fruits, vegetables, beans, and whole grains are excellent sources of fiber.

How It Works

By increasing the weight of stools, fiber puts pressure on the colon to empty. This helps prevent constipation. The two kinds of fiber are insoluble fiber, which can't be broken down at all, and soluble fiber, which dissolves in water. Most fibrous foods contain both types of fiber. Insoluble fiber—found in soaked or sprouted seeds or nuts, broccoli, cauliflower, carrots, celery, and lettuce—is believed to reduce the risk of colorectal cancer, although scientists aren't sure why. One theory is that the increased weight of stools hurries waste matter though the colon and reduces the amount of time that carcinogens remain in the body. Another theory is that fiber reduces concentrations of caustic fecal bile acids.

Some studies suggest that a diet high in fiber helps prevent peptic ulcer disease and reduces the likelihood of a duodenal ulcer relapsing. Why fiber helps prevent a peptic ulcer is also still an open question. One theory is that fibrous food travels faster through the gastrointestinal tract, so the GI tract is not as exposed to ulcer-causing acid.

How To Use

Eat fruit or a vegetable with every meal. Not only do these foods contain fiber, but they are full of vitamins and minerals, and they are not fattening. Fruit makes an excellent snack food as well.

Cautions

Fibrous foods that contain water are the best sources of fiber, because with these foods you don't run the risk of getting bezoar formation—a large concentration of dry food—that blocks the gastrointestinal tract. Oatmeal and vegetable soup are excellent sources of fiber because they contain water. Fruits such as oranges, apples, and pineapples, which contain water, are also recommended. Granola bars, bran, immoderate amounts of wheat bread, and fibrous crackers are not as good a source of fiber as their manufacturers claim because they don't contain water. Dry fibrous foods can be extremely irritating to people who have gastrointestinal problems.

Mastic Gum

Mastic gum, sometimes called mastika, is a resinous extract made from the stems and leaves of the Greek pistachio tree (*Pistacia lentiscus*). Much anecdotal evidence exists for mastic gum being useful against peptic disorders. In Greece, where it is chewed, or masticated, after meals, mastic gum is a folk remedy for heartburn, abdominal pains, dyspepsia, and gastric ulcers. The lemony, balsam-scented gum is also an ingredient in Greek cuisine. Most of the world's production of mastic gum comes from the *Mastichochoria*, the "mastic villages" located in the southern part of the Greek island of Chios. Mastic gum is easily tolerated and has no side effects.

How It Works

Several studies on the effect of mastic gum on gastric ulcers have been performed, and the studies have shown positive, albeit inconclusive, results. In a double-blind study of thirty-eight patients with duodenal ulcers, 80 percent of patients who took one gram per day of mastic gum saw a reduction in ulcer symptoms, whereas only 50 percent of patients who took a placebo saw reductions. In the study, researchers used an endoscope to examine patients' duodenal tissue, and they reported healing in 70 percent of mastic-gum patients but only 22 percent of placebo patients. Another study looked at gastric and duodenal ulcers in rats and found that oral doses, roughly the equivalent of 500 mg per day in humans, reduced both gastric acid secretions and damage to the stomach lining.

In 1998, researchers at University Hospital in Nottingham, England, conducted a very interesting study in which they demonstrated that mastic gum kills *H. pylori,* the bacterium that causes ulcers. They wrote, "Even low doses of mastic gum—1 gram per day for 2 weeks—can cure peptic ulcers very rapidly." However, the *H. pylori* bacteria killed in this experiment died in the test tube. The stomach is a delicately balanced and extremely complex environment—far more complex than any environment a scientist could create in a test tube. The question remains whether commercially available mastic gum supplements can match the results of this *in vitro* experiment and really kill or alter *H. pylori.*

How To Use

The recommended dose of mastic gum is 250 to 500 mg taken fifteen minutes before every meal and two hours before bedtime.

Cautions

There are no known cases of sensitivities or allergies to mastic gum.

Vitamin C

Vitamin C reduces the severity of colds, awakens the immune system, and prevents secondary viral and bacterial infections. It is also one of nature's most potent antioxidants. An antioxidant is a molecule capable, to a certain extent, of reversing the damage that free radicals do to body tissue. A free radical is a very unstable, highly reactive molecule with an unpaired electron. Because electrons want to occur in pairs, unpaired free radicals steal electrons from other molecules. This process is called oxidation. Oxidation can damage cell membranes and DNA. It can damage tissue and accelerate the aging process. To see oxidation with your own eyes, cut an apple in half and observe it an hour later. The brown decay on the inside of the apple is caused by oxidation. An antioxidant is a substance that reverses this decay by deactivating unstable free radicals. Vitamin A, vitamin C, vitamin E, and selenium (or ACES, as they are sometimes collectively called) are the most potent antioxidants.

How It Works

Some have proposed that a deficiency of antioxidants makes the stomach and duodenum more susceptible to infection by *H. pylori* bacteria. Given that vitamin C is an antioxidant, several studies have been undertaken to see if vitamin C is useful against *H. pylori* infections.

Scientists in Poland conducted a study comparing antacids and high doses of vitamin C for the treatment of *H. pylori* infections. In the study, fifty-one *H. pylori*-infected patients suffering from chronic gastritis took either antacid tablets or 5 g—yes, 5 *grams!*—of vitamin C daily for four weeks. Vitamin C levels in the patients' gastric juice were measured at the start, middle, and end of the study. In the vitamin C group, the bacterium was eradicated in eight of twenty-seven patients, and gastric juice vitamin C concentrations rose significantly. In the antacid group, all patients remained infected with *H. pylori*, and vitamin C gastric juice concentrations remained the same.

A study by researchers at the San Francisco VA Medical Center of stored blood samples from 6,746 adults found that white people with lower levels of vitamin C in their blood are more likely to be infected by *H. pylori* bacteria. This data indicates that blood vitamin C levels may determine a person's risk of being infected by *H. pylori*, although it could be that being infected with the bacteria lowers vitamin C levels in the blood. In ethnic minorities, low vitamin C blood levels did not indicate a higher risk of being infected by *H. pylori*.

Swedish scientists conducted an experiment in which they administered vitamin C, the microalga *Haematococcus pluvialis* (it is high in vitamin C), or a non-vitamin C meal to *H. pylori*-infected mice for ten days. The scientists then dissected the mice and examined their stomachs. Mice who had taken vitamin C or the alga meal "showed significantly lower colonization levels and lower inflammation scores" than the other mice. Moreover, the vitamin C and alga meal inhibited *H. pylori* growth in test-tube experiments.

How To Use

The best way to take vitamin C is to get it from citrus fruit, strawberries, kiwi, spinach, broccoli, collard greens, potatoes, and tomatoes. The body recognizes and absorbs the vitamin C in those foods. Most vitamin C above the amount of 500 mg is excreted in the urine without bringing any benefit. Most people have had the experience of taking vitamin C tablets and noticing their discolored urine. For this reason, vitamin C has been called "expensive urine."

Cautions

Some physicians do not recommend taking so-called megadoses of vitamin C (500 mg or more) on a daily basis. A 2001 study conducted by researchers at the University of Pennsylvania suggested that very large doses of vitamin C could cause, not prevent, oxidative damage to DNA in cells. Another study suggested that megadoses of vitamin C could cause hardening of the arteries.

If you have a sensitive bowel—if you have irritable bowel syndrome, for example—do not take vitamin C supplements. Vitamin C has been known to cause immediate diarrhea in people who have sensitive bowels.

MYTHS AND "OLD WIVES' TALES" ABOUT ULCER HEALING

I thought it would be a good idea to shoot down a couple of myths concerning herbs that are supposed to heal ulcers. In popular literature, garlic and jalapeño peppers are sometimes mentioned as agents that are capable of healing ulcers. I looked into it and found that this is not true. Here's another surprise: Milk, contrary to what grandma said, is good for neither ulcers nor heartburn.

Garlic

Garlic, or the stinking rose (as it is known to chefs who like to use it in their concoctions), is an antioxidant and a preventative against the common cold. Garlic has antifungal properties, as well. It may even be useful as an insect repellant. As far back as 1848, Louis Pasteur demonstrated how allyl, a substance derived from garlic, could kill bacteria. But can garlic kill *H. pylori,* the bacterium that causes peptic ulcers?

The answer appears to be no. Confirming the results of a study on jalapeño peppers and garlic (see "Jalapeño Peppers" below), scientists in Germany conducted a study in which twenty *H. pylori*-infected people were given 300 mg of dried garlic powder for eight weeks. Urea breath tests given after the eight-week period revealed that only one patient was no longer infected. In fairness to fans of garlic, I should point out that critics of this study maintain that the researchers should have used fresh crushed garlic instead of the dried powder. Only fresh garlic, the critics maintain, has quantities of allicin potent enough to kill *H. pylori* bacteria. Allicin is the oily yellow liquid that gives garlic its pungent odor and flavor.

Jalapeño Peppers

Given how hot jalapeño peppers are and how much they sting the mouth and throat, the idea that jalapeño peppers can prevent stomach ulcers seems incredible—and it is incredible. In some parts of the world, however, jalapeño peppers are a folk remedy for ulcers.

In the test tube, the capsaicin in jalapeño peppers—the crystalline alkaloid that is responsible for the pepper's heat—has been shown to kill *H. pylori,* the bacteria that cause ulcers. To test whether jalapeño peppers can kill *H. pylori* in human stomachs as well as test tubes, researchers at the Baylor College of Medicine fed twelve *H. pylori*-infected adults beef, tortillas, and salad along with ten garlic gloves, six sliced jalapeño peppers, bismuth tablets, or nothing at all. The subjects of this tasty experiment were given before-and-after urea breath tests to find out whether the food they ate or tablets they took affected the bacterial levels in their stomachs. Unfortunately, neither the jalapeño peppers nor the garlic had any effect. The bismuth, however, had a "marked inhibitory effect" on *H. pylori* levels. Even jalapeño peppers, it appears, are no match for hardy *H. pylori* bacteria.

Milk

Milk is a folk remedy for ulcers, heartburn, and dyspepsia in many parts of the world. In the United States, people with heartburn and indigestion sometimes drink a glass of warm milk before going to bed.

In the short term, milk relieves ulcer pain because it temporarily coats the ulcer sore and prevents it from being irritated by gastric acid. Milk, however, also stimulates the production of gastric acid. Actually, milk stimulates hydrochloric acid production to roughly the same degree as beer and wine. In the long term, drinking milk actually irritates an ulcer and causes more ulcer pain, because milk subjects the ulcer to more gastric acid. In a study called "Relative stimulatory effects of commonly ingested beverages on gastric acid secretion in humans," K. McArthur et al. demonstrated that milk is on par with wine and beer when it comes to the secretion of gastric acid in the stomach. This book is by no means prejudiced against folk remedies, but you would do well to avoid this particular folk remedy if you have an ulcer.

EXERCISE

At the turn of the twentieth century, the Physical Culture Movement was all the rage in Germany and the United States. Its guiding principle was simple: A physically fit body produces good health. Throughout both countries, health sanitariums were founded to educate the public and cure various afflictions, including peptic ulcers. While these spa-like facilities professed to have perfected their own interesting programs, their common denominator was exercise, and plenty of it.

How It Works

According to a recent study published in the *Western Journal of Medicine,* exercising decreases a man's chances of getting a duodenal ulcer (although not a stomach ulcer). In the study, researchers looked at the exercise habits of 11,413 men who attended the Cooper Institute for Aerobics Research between 1970 and 1990. Compared with sedentary men, men who ran ten miles or more per week were 62 percent less likely to acquire duodenal ulcers, while men who ran ten miles or less were 50 percent less likely. Why were the running men not as subject to duodenal ulcers? Running may have strengthened their immune systems, helped them cope with stress, or perhaps reduced the production of acid in their digestive tracts.

How To Use

Whatever type of exercise you choose, the most import thing is to exercise regularly. One hour a day is recommended; if you exercise at a gym and can take advantage of the different exercise machines, you get a better workout, and I recommend doing such an exercise regimen three times a week at least. People who exercise only once a week do not get the benefit of exercise. Regularity is the key.

Cautions

Before starting any rigorous form of exercise program, make sure to have a complete physical checkup. The older you are, the more important this rule becomes. If everything checks out, start off your program in small increments. Initially, never push yourself to the point of exhaustion, even if your test results are fine. Build up your stamina as you learn to know and appreciate your body's limits.

TRADITIONAL CHINESE MEDICINE TREATMENTS

Traditional Chinese Medicine (TCM) is very different from conventional western medicine. It has been said that Traditional Chinese Medicine attempts to understand the body as an ecosystem or single component in nature. Whereas a western doctor studies a symptom in order to determine the underlying disease, a Chinese doctor sees the symptom as part of a totality. Western medicine is concerned with isolating diseases in order to treat them. TCM seeks to remedy a "pattern of disharmony," or imbalance, in the patient.

The principles of Traditional Chinese Medicine can be found in Taoism, the ancient philosophy or religion in which the practitioner strives to follow the correct path, or Tao, and thereby find a rightful place in the universe. Taoists believe that the universe is animated by an omnipresent life-energy called *Qi* (pronounced CHEE). Qi, meanwhile, comprises two primal opposites, *yin* and *yang*. The yin and yang complement each other and are always interacting. In a healthy human body, Qi circulates unimpeded and the balance of yin and yang is maintained. But an excess of yin or yang, or a blockage of Qi, can create a pattern of disharmony and render the patient ill (the premise behind acupuncture is that the needles unblock Qi energy). As such, no disease has a cause, according to Traditional Chinese Medicine. Rather, disease is a malevolent configuration of yin-yang forces in the body.

In Traditional Chinese Medicine, peptic ulcers are usually treated with a combination of the following herbs:

- **Cat's claw *(Uncaria tomentosa).*** This herb is known for its anti-inflammatory properties.

- **Danshen (*Salvia miltiorrhiza*).** Traditionally used in China to treat abdominal pain, this herb also improves circulation.

- **Meadowsweet (*Filipendula ulmaria*).** Traditionally used in China to treat peptic ulcers and indigestion.

Your Traditional Chinese Medicine practitioner will tell you how to take these herbs and in what quantity.

From 1999 until 2002, I was a visiting professor at the school of (Traditional) Chinese Medicine at the University of Hong Kong. My task was to bring a scientific, western method of evaluation to a number of Traditional Chinese Medicines. My colleagues and I determined that the problems with Chinese medicines are as follows:

- The selection of the herbs is rarely known. We could never be entirely certain which herbs we were dealing with.

- The source of herbs is difficult to trace.

- A structural analysis of herbs is not required by law or proffered by the manufacturers, and unless you do a structural analysis on your own, you can't be sure which chemicals are in an herb.

- Until recently, clinical studies conducted on the herbs in China were poorly done with little attention paid to protocols. The studies were not controlled and did not include placebo data.

• The herbs included high amounts of heavy metals.

Basically, whatever herb or herbs your practitioner of Traditional Chinese Medicine recommends for you, you should obtain the herbs from an American supplier. Unlike Chinese suppliers, American suppliers offer organic, standardized ingredients. Most American suppliers comply with good manufacturing practices.

CONCLUSION

Interestingly enough, many of the remedies described above provide an easy means of preventing peptic ulcers from ever forming. A number of them also provide ways of easing the painful symptoms of this condition. And a few show promise of helping reverse the problem. So if you are looking for a safe natural approach to avoiding ulcers or reducing the symptoms of ulcers, this chapter may be just what the doctor ordered. On the other hand, if you are looking for a quick cure, scientifically speaking, the jury is still out.

More work needs to be done to scientifically prove any of these alternative approaches as effective or superior to those treatments discussed in the previous chapter. There is, however, growing evidence that a relatively new nutrient—the result of a simple combination of molecules—has been developed to bridge the gap between alternative and conventional therapies. You will learn more about this breakthrough in the next chapter.

8

A Natural Approach to Ulcer Treatment

As a scientist, I am always astonished by the advancements medical researchers are making in the development of life-saving drugs. As a physician, I clearly understand the public's growing interest in natural remedies that enable the body to heal itself. And as a teacher, I can't help but tell people about a treatment that combines a natural approach to healing and is grounded in actual scientific research. Zinc-Carnosine is just such a breakthrough.

Having had a long-standing interest in the treatment of ulcers, as I pointed out in the book's Introduction, I was made aware of Zinc-Carnosine several years ago. Because of my position as a visiting professor at the University of Hong Kong's medical school, I was fortunate enough to come across a number of reports on Zinc-Carnosine. The scientific literature seemed very credible. As it turns out, Zinc-Carnosine has had remarkable success in Japan as a treatment for peptic ulcer disease, but the supplement is hardly known in North America and Europe. Hopefully, this book will change that.

Zinc-Carnosine deserves consideration as a first-line ulcer treatment in this part of the world. Besides ulcers, Zinc-Carnosine is valuable for treating gastritis and dyspepsia. The supplement represents a natural healing approach to stomach ailments. Instead of obstructing an action of the stomach—blocking acid production, neutralizing hydrochloric acid—Zinc-Carnosine strengthens the stomach's mucosal defenses. The supplement harnesses the stomach's natural ability to fight disease, battle infection, and heal itself.

This chapter explains what Zinc-Carnosine is and examines whether it is safe. I look at how the supplement heals ulcers and relieves ulcer pain. In the second half of this chapter, I examine the science behind Zinc-Carnosine. I will cite many studies that show how Zinc-Carnosine achieves its healing power. However, let's start at the beginning, and look at zinc and L-carnosine—the two components of Zinc-Carnosine— separately.

WHAT IS ZINC?

Zinc, an essential mineral, is found in almost every body cell. Zinc is important for the functioning of the immune system. It is a component of many enzymes and necessary for DNA synthesis. Of interest to this discussion, zinc plays a role in wound healing. It is involved in the thymus gland's production of T-lymphocytes, the white blood cells that manage the response of the immune system to an injury or infection (the *T* in T-lymphocyte stands for "thymus"). People with zinc deficiencies heal poorly because their immune systems are impaired. As a measure of how important zinc is to healing, a controlled study published in the *Annals of Surgery* found that the healing time of surgical wounds was reduced by 43 percent when patients took 220 mg of zinc sulfate three times daily. Oysters are the best natural source of zinc. The mineral is also found in beef, pork, seafood, beans, and nuts. Many breakfast cereals are fortified with zinc.

WHAT IS L-CARNOSINE?

L-carnosine is a dipeptide bond composed of two essential amino acids, L-histidine and beta-alanine. Amino acids are the material from which protein is made. L-carnosine demonstrates antioxidant properties. It occurs naturally in the cells of all mammals, so taking L-carnosine does not introduce any foreign substances into your body. You can obtain L-carnosine by including meat and beans in your regular diet.

The L-histidine part of the L-carnosine dipeptide is interesting because histidine is the precursor of histamine, and, as Chapter 6 explains, histamine plays a role in the production of hydrochloric acid in the stomach. A precursor is a substance that precedes, and is necessary for, the creation of another substance. It could be that the L-histidine creates histamine that in some way controls or modulates the stomach's production of hydrochloric acid.

ZINC-CARNOSINE

When zinc and L-carnosine are chemically joined, a unique nutrient is formed. It is called Zinc-Carnosine. It is insoluble in water and heat-stable. Why is this important? First, because it doesn't dissolve in water, it doesn't easily lose its potency, nor is it quickly flushed out of the body. And second, being heat-stable, hot and cold temperatures will not change its ability to work. The supplement's heat-stability gives the pills and tablets a long shelf-life.

The peptic-ulcer healing rate from Zinc-Carnosine, as observed by endoscopy, is approximately 65 percent after the standard eight-week treatment. The improvement, in terms of symptoms and other objective criteria, is about 70 percent. Zinc-Carnosine is the first anti-ulcer drug to include zinc, a substance known for its healing properties. How Zinc-Carnosine works is explained throughout this chapter. Meanwhile, here is what Zinc-Carnosine does in a nutshell. This nutrient:

- Protects the membranes of epithelial cells in the stomach and brings the cells back to their normal metabolism.

- Acts as an antioxidant.

- Has anti-inflammatory properties.

- Adheres to stomach ulcer sores and acts as a barrier between the sores and caustic gastric juice.

- After adhering to sores, releases its zinc and L-carnosine for healing purposes.

- Has an inhibitory effect on *H. pylori* bacteria.

- Is prostaglandin-independent and doesn't interfere with the prostaglandin production that is necessary for the stomach's mucosal protection.

Patients taking Zinc-Carnosine have reported no significant

adverse effects or side effects. The supplement does not cause zinc toxicity or interfere with the absorption of copper, which is a concern whenever zinc is ingested.

Zinc-Carnosine was developed in the late 1980s by Hamari Ltd. of Osaka in Japan. Since 1994, it has been in widespread clinical use in Japan, where it is known under the generic name polaprezinc. Based upon scientific data supplied by the Japanese medical researchers, the inventors at Hamari took out a complete line of patents in the United States, Canada, and Europe. The first U.S. patent, 4,981,846, was issued in 1991 and covered the composition of the Zinc-Carnosine molecule and its anti-ulcer activity. Several more patents soon followed, but Zinc-Carnosine was not developed commercially until it was submitted to the Food and Drug Administration as a new dietary ingredient (NDI) in May 2002. After completing the review process in late 2002, Zinc-Carnosine was made available as a supplement in the United States.

Ingredients of Zinc-Carnosine

Zinc-Carnosine is a chelated—a chemically joined—compound that combines the trace mineral zinc and L-carnosine. Chelated compounds are firmly attached, which is an advantage in the digestive system where hydrochloric acid and pepsin readily break down everything that comes their way. On their own, zinc and L-carnosine soon disassociate in the stomach's acidic environment, but, owing to its chelated structure, the Zinc–L-carnosine compound doesn't disassociate as easily. This accounts for Zinc-Carnosine's staying power in the stomach. Both zinc and L-carnosine have healing properties in their own right, but, as numerous experiments have demonstrated, the compounded healing effect of the two ingredients is much greater than that of zinc or L-carnosine on its own. As a compound, zinc and L-carnosine make for a dynamic healing agent. Zinc-Carnosine is much greater than the sum of its parts.

How Zinc-Carnosine Heals Ulcers

Zinc-Carnosine relieves stomach pain, heals ulcers, and perhaps prevents them. How? The supplement works by strengthening the

What Is Chelation?

Chelation is the chemical bonding or attaching together of two different molecules. Chelation is quite different from physically mixing different component parts. By chelating two components, you can slow their absorption as nutrients. Chelation is often associated with essential minerals. We need essential minerals for nutrition, but their consumption can have uncomfortable side effects. The consumption of zinc by itself, for example, can cause nausea. Chelation causes essential minerals to release their molecules slowly, and, therefore, be tolerated better by the body. Because the slow release makes the molecules easier to absorb, bonding minerals by chelation is the preferred method.

stomach mucosa, sticking to the stomach wall and acting as a buffer to gastric acid, serving as an antioxidant, controlling the inflammatory response to stomach injury, and inhibiting the growth of *H. pylori* bacteria. You'll learn more about each of these important actions directly below, and will discover the technical details of Zinc-Carnosine's mode of action later in the chapter.

Strengthens the Stomach Mucosa

The lining of the stomach is protected from its own caustic gastric juice by a thin gel-like layer of mucus. When this mucus layer erodes, the stomach lining is exposed, and you can get an ulcer. Evidence suggests that Zinc-Carnosine works primarily by strengthening the mucosal barrier between the stomach lining and the harsh gastric juices of the stomach. The supplement appears to adhere to the stomach wall to provide protection to all areas of the stomach. These studies give a picture of Zinc-Carnosine's protective effect on the stomach lining:

- In an early study conducted at the Yokohama Red Cross Hospital in 1992, twenty-five patients whose ulcers were confirmed by endoscopy were given 75 mg Zinc-Carnosine tablets twice daily (one after breakfast and one before bed) for eight weeks. Drugs such as H_2 blockers and proton pump inhibitors that might affect the results of the study were prohibited. The "disappearance rate" of epigastric pain symptoms in the patients was 53.3 percent after meals, 76.9 percent fasting, and 90.9 percent at night. Of the twenty-five subjects who had a final assessment by endoscopy after the eight weeks, 65 percent were healed of their gastric ulcers. This study is interesting because the ulcers were healed without suppressing the production of acid. Zinc-Carnosine was able to provide a genuine protective effect to the stomach.

- In a double-blind study of three groups taking 50-mg, 75-mg, or 100-mg Zinc-Carnosine tablets twice daily for eight weeks, the success rates of the study as obtained by endoscopy were as follows: 50.8 percent for 100-mg group, 58.6 percent for 150-mg group, and 53.6 percent for 200-mg group.

These studies show very clearly that Zinc-Carnosine has a protective effect on the stomach, and that the supplement's healing action is not based solely on its role as a buffer of stomach acid.

Adheres to the Stomach Wall

Like bismuth and to a lesser degree sucralfate, Zinc-Carnosine coats the stomach and acts as a barrier between ulcers and hydrochloric acid. In this way, it protects ulcer sores from irritation by acid, relieves pain, and permits the sores to heal. In a 1992 study called "The gastric mucosal adhesiveness of Z-103 (Zinc-Carnosine) in rats with chronic ulcer," M. Seiki et al. concluded, "(Zinc-Carnosine) shows a long-term adhesive and permeable action on the gastric mucosa in acetic acid ulcer rats, and it has a comparable high affinity at the ulcerous site." The scientists attributed Zinc-Carnosine's adhesiveness to its zinc content. They also noted that the strength and duration of adhesiveness was dose-dependent, which indicates that Zinc-Carnosine has a genuine adhesive effect in the stomach.

Acts as an Antioxidant

More so than most other organs, the stomach is subject to oxidative stress from alcohol, swallowed tobacco smoke or juice, and other harmful substances. Zinc-Carnosine acts as an antioxidant to prevent these substances from eroding the stomach lining. I describe experiments involving Zinc-Carnosine and its antioxidant properties in the second half of this chapter.

Tempers the Inflammatory Process

Inflammation is a natural response of the immune system to injury. Nevertheless, too much inflammation in the stomach can cause gastritis and painful ulcers. In experiments, the supplement Zinc-Carnosine retarded the TNF-alpha secretion of interleukin-8, a molecule involved in the inflammatory process. The supplement therefore appears to modulate the immune-system response and keep inflammation in check.

Inhibits H. Pylori

H. pylori bacteria are responsible for seventy-five percent of stomach ulcers worldwide. Zinc-Carnosine inhibits the growth of the bacteria, probably by strengthening the stomach mucosa and making it less susceptible to a bacterial infection.

Other Indications of Zinc-Carnosine

The digestive tract is a continuum. Although each organ plays a specific role in absorption and digestion, the organs don't begin and end abruptly. If you were to take sequential tissue biopsies throughout the digestive tract, you would see that there is a steady, gradual transition from one organ to the next. Each organ has its epithelium and sublayer that supports the epithelium. The mechanisms of cell survival and protection are the same throughout. It stands to reason, therefore, that a drug or supplement that is good for one part of the GI tract can also be good for another part.

Because Zinc-Carnosine heals ulcers in the stomach, scientists at Medical School Hospital, Sendagi, Tokyo, decided to see if it could be used effectively to treat mouth ulcers and stomatitis, the inflammation of the lining of the mouth. For the experiment, rats' cheek pouches were injected with an acetic acid solution. After lesions formed, they were injected daily with either Zinc-Carnosine or water. Beginning on the seventh day of the experiment, lesions injected with Zinc-Carnosine healed significantly better. The scientists also examined the mucous membrane in the rats' cheek pouches and found, in the Zinc-Carnosine group, that the thickening of the mucous membrane was less severe.

This experiment shows that Zinc-Carnosine may be useful, for example, for healing the stomatitis that often results from chemotherapy. Perhaps scientists in the years to come will find other ways to put Zinc-Carnosine to use. For instance, the supplement is now being investigated as a sunscreen. Moreover, Zinc-Carnosine may be osteogenic, meaning that it builds bones, and therefore could be a treatment option for osteoporosis.

Studies – Modes of Action

We know that Zinc-Carnosine works to relieve stomach pain, heal ulcers, and perhaps prevent ulcers. For scientists, however, the major question is never *what*, but *how* and *why*. How does Zinc-Carnosine relieve stomach pain and heal ulcers? Since it was invented in the early 1990s, Zinc-Carnosine has been the subject of several dozen studies, most of them conducted in Japan, where ulcer patients have been taking the supplement for a decade. In the remainder of this chapter, I look at studies that I believe reveal the most about Zinc-Carnosine's healing action. Of the numerous studies conducted on Zinc-Carnosine, I selected those studies that were conducted exceptionally well, or that examined a particular mode of healing action. The studies reveal the how and the why of Zinc-Carnosine.

The study of Zinc-Carnosine is still in its infancy. There is much that we don't know, but I believe that Zinc-Carnosine ranks with bismuth and proton pump inhibitors as a therapy for treating ulcer disease. I predict that the supplement will become a standard option for treating ulcers in the years ahead. As the supplement gains in popularity, it will no doubt become the subject of more studies, and the coming decade will probably bring to light much that we don't yet know about the healing action of Zinc-Carnosine.

Antioxidant Effect

Oxidation damages DNA, cell membranes, and tissue. It is caused by very unstable, highly reactive molecules called free radicals that steal electrons from other molecules. An antioxidant is a substance that reverses this decay by deactivating unstable free radicals. In a study conducted at the Zeria Pharmaceutical in Japan, researchers Y. Hori et al. looked at the effect of Zinc-Carnosine as an antioxidant. In the test tube, the researchers discovered that Zinc-Carnosine scavenged active-oxygen free-radical species, including hydrogen peroxide. This free radical is produced in the stomach and elsewhere in the body to kill pathogens. In the stomach, however, it can also attack and erode the stomach lining. By scavenging and destroying hydrogen-peroxide free radicals, Zinc-Carnosine protected stomach cells in test-tube experiments. The scientists also conducted experiments with Zinc-Carnosine on rats by inducing ischemia in the rats' stomachs and exposing the rats to 200-proof alcohol. Ischemia is a condition in which blood flow to a part of the body is constricted. The alcohol and lack of blood created massive oxidative stress in the rats' stomachs, but the scientists discovered that free radical scavenging by Zinc-Carnosine inhibited the damage created by ischemia and alcohol in a dose-dependent way. In other words, damage was reduced according to the amount of Zinc-Carnosine fed to the rats. This is important because it showed that Zinc-Carnosine had a genuine protective antioxidant effect on the rats' injured stomachs.

In a similar study conducted at Dokkyo University School of Medicine in Japan, H. Hiraishi et al. looked at the antioxidant effect of Zinc-Carnosine on stomach cells in the test tube. This study was interesting because it involved cytochrome C, a protein found in cells. Normally, cytochrome C figures in the creation of cellular energy, but when a cell is damaged, it releases cytochrome C into its mitochondria, and this triggers cell apoptosis, the programmed self-destruction, or death, of the cell. Scientists can measure the release of cytochrome C from cells to get a better understanding of how noxious agents such as alcohol affect cells. If the cells release sufficient amounts of cytochrome C, it indicates that they are being damaged. For the experiment, researchers cultured cells from the fundus (the convex upper portion) of rats' stomachs. Then, in the test tube, they exposed the cells to hydrogen peroxide and 200-proof alcohol, as well as various amounts of Zinc-Carnosine, and measured the cells' release of cytochrome C. The purpose of the experiment was to see if Zinc-Carnosine, as measured by the release of cytochrome C, could prevent cell damage. The scientists found that Zinc-Carnosine inhibited the release of cytochrome C from the cells in a dose-dependent manner. In other words, the more Zinc-Carnosine that was applied to a cell, the less likely it was to be damaged by alcohol and hydrogen peroxide. This excellent experiment clearly demonstrates that Zinc-Carnosine can protect stomach cells from damage by alcohol and other noxious substances.

Inflammatory Response

Inflammation is a natural response on the part of the immune system to injuries and infections. When you sprain your ankle, for example, redness, warmth, and swelling occur at the site of the injury. In other words, inflammation occurs. Swelling and redness are the result of blood vessels dilating at the site of the injury so that more blood can arrive and bathe the injury with white blood cells and other healing agents. Warmth is meant to kill bacteria and toxins. The problem with inflammation of this kind is that it can create problems in its own right. In the stomach, inflammation can cause gastritis. Ulcers can appear where tissue is inflamed. And inflammation, of course, is painful.

In the nucleus of certain kinds of cells are molecules that create inflammation. These molecules include interleukin-8 (IL-8). Interleukins are molecules that help white blood cells communicate with one another. In gastric mucosal cells, IL-8 plays a major role in the inflammatory response to an *H. pylori* infection. Because sustained inflammation is a risk for gastric mucosal damage, agents that down-regulate the inflammatory response—agents that retard the effect of IL-8 and decrease inflammation—may be useful for treating *H. pylori* infections.

In a study conducted at Dokkyo University School of Medicine in Japan by T. Shimada et al., scientists performed an experiment to see whether Zinc-Carnosine down-regulates IL-8 and thereby controls the inflammatory response of gastric mucosal cells to an *H. pylori* infection. Because a molecule called NF-kappaB stimulates the production of IL-8, the scientists also examined the effect of Zinc-Carnosine on NF-kappaB activity. The experiment was undertaken with an enzyme-linked immunosorbent assay (ELISA) and an electrophoretic mobility shift assay kit—two means of identifying and quantifying proteins, in this case IL-8 and NF-kappaB.

The scientists found that Zinc-Carnosine suppressed the IL-8 secretion of TNF-alpha (tumor necrosis factor-alpha), a powerful substance that creates inflammation, in a dose-dependent manner. The more Zinc-Carnosine administered, the less TNF-alpha produced. The supplement also suppressed NF-kappaB. This experiment has implications for the treatment of *H. pylori*-induced ulcers with Zinc-Carnosine. Zinc-Carnosine may be a good candidate to serve along with antibiotics in triple and quadruple therapies for the eradication of *H. pylori*. (These drug therapies are explained in Chapter 6.) In any case, the supplement appears to retard the inflammatory process, which helps in the prevention of ulcers and gastritis.

One point I've made in this book—and I'm sorry if I've been hammering at it too obsessively—is that peptic ulcer disease caused by the use of NSAIDs is on the rise, and that doctors need to find ways of treating ulcers in patients who must keep taking NSAIDs for their osteoporosis or arthritis pain. The following experiment is most interesting because it addressed this problem head on. It examined the effect of Zinc-Carnosine on aspirin-induced gastric mucosal injury. For the experiment, which was conducted at the Kyoto Prefectural University of Medicine by Y Naito et al., scientists pretreated rats with Zinc-Carnosine, and then, with a catheter, poured acidified aspirin into the rats' stomachs. This caused acute inflammation and hemorrhaging ulcers, although the size of the gastric erosions was significantly inhibited in a dose-dependent manner by Zinc-Carnosine. Oxidative stress and the gastric concentration of tumor necrosis factor-alpha (TNF-alpha) were also inhibited in a dose-dependent manner. TNF-alpha, a cytokine, is involved in the inflammatory response.

This experiment suggests that Zinc-Carnosine, as well as being an antioxidant, modulates the immune-system response to prevent inflammation in the stomach caused by NSAIDs.

Human Insulin-Like Growth Factor 1 (IGF-1)

Human insulin-like growth factor 1 (IGF-1), a polypeptide, is involved in the growth and development of muscle, fat, brain, and bone cells. It acts as a stimulating hormone in protein synthesis. IGF-1 mimics some of the metabolic actions of insulin. For example, it makes cells healthier by stimulating the uptake of glucose and amino acids. Besides increasing the production of mucus in the stomach and acting as an antioxidant, Zinc-Carnosine may also heal gastric epithelial cells by stimulating the production of IGF-1.

To test this theory, scientists at Kyoto Pharmaceutical University in Kyoto, Japan led by S. Kato et al., performed an experiment on two groups of rats. First, they injected an adjuvant in one group to induce arthritis. Then they induced stomach ulcers in both groups. Rats in each group were treated with either omeprazole, a proton pump inhibitor, or Zinc-Carnosine for fourteen days. The scientists used arthritic rats for their experiment because arthritis is known to decrease the production of IGF-1 in the gastric mucosa. By comparing ulcer-healing rates in the arthritic and nonarthritic rats, they could study how much of a role Zinc-Carnosine plays in the production of IGF-1. In other words, they could discover if Zinc-Carnosine heals ulcers in part by increasing IGF-1 production. This experiment also served as a comparison between Zinc-Carnosine and the proton pump inhibitor omeprazole.

Overall, ulcers in the arthritic rats healed more slowly than ulcers in the nonarthritic rats. Both omeprazole and Zinc-Carnosine increased the healing rates of arthritic rats, although, wrote the authors, the "omeprazole action is mainly due to the inhibition of acid secretion, while the polaprezinc (Zinc-Carnosine) effect, as shown in the study, may be ascribed mainly to the stimulation of IGF-1." The scientists judged the healing effect of Zinc-Carnosine on arthritic rats "more pronounced" than that of omeprazole. This experiment was especially interesting because it applies to arthritic humans as well as arthritic rats. People with arthritis must take

NSAIDs to relieve the accompanying pain, and taking NSAIDs increases their chances of getting an ulcer. This experiment shows that Zinc-Carnosine may well be an excellent treatment for ulcer patients who must continue taking NSAIDs for their arthritis, because the supplement stimulates the production of IGF-1.

In a similar experiment conducted at Kyoto Pharmaceutical University, scientists tested Zinc-Carnosine on diabetic rats. These rats, of course, lack insulin. The object of the experiment was to determine if Zinc-Carnosine could stimulate the production of insulin-like growth factor 1, and, in so doing, work to heal the rats' ulcers. For the experiment, rats were injected with streptozotocin, a substance that destroys the cells in the pancreas that create insulin. Five weeks later, the newly diabetic rats' blood glucose levels (BGLs) were above 350 mg/100 ml, more than three times higher than the normal level. They were given insulin to keep them alive, hydrochloric acid to induce ulcers, and, twice daily for four days, Zinc-Carnosine (3-30 mg/kg) or one of its components, zinc or L-carnosine. Under the influence of Zinc-Carnosine, the rats' ulcers healed within ten days without affecting glucose levels or acid secretion. Zinc had a similar, but not as pronounced effect, on healing rates, but L-carnosine did not heal the rats' ulcers. The scientists attributed Zinc-Carnosine's healing power to augmented IGF-1 synthesis in the rats' stomach mucosa. It appears that IGF-1 stimulation is indeed an important part of Zinc-Carnosine's mode of action in the stomach.

An interesting experiment conducted by K. Seto et al. of the Zeria Pharmaceutical Company in Saitama, Japan, also attempted to clarify the ulcer-healing properties of Zinc-Carnosine. For the experiment, the scientists compared the effect of Zinc-Carnosine, as well as zinc by itself and L-carnosine by itself, on fibroblast cells from humans, endothelial cells from humans, and mucosal epithelial cells from guinea pigs' stomachs. The goal of the experiment was to find out how Zinc-Carnosine achieves its healing power in tissue. The scientists were especially curious to compare the effect of Zinc-Carnosine, zinc alone, and L-carnosine alone on cell growth and proliferation. As part of the experiment, they also looked at the effect of Zinc-Carnosine on the production of human insulin-like growth factor 1 (IGF-1). As I explained earlier, this molecule is involved in the growth and development of cells. Studies have shown that blood concentrations of IGF-1 are low in zinc-deficient rats, and the scientists wanted to discover if the zinc component of Zinc-Carnosine stimulates the production of IGF-1.

Here are the results of the experiment:

- Zinc-Carnosine stimulated the growth and proliferation of human endothelial and fibroblast cells, but had no effect on mucosal epithelial cells from guinea pigs' stomachs. Endothelial cells line the heart and blood vessels. Fibroblast cells are found in collagen, the substance that forms the structural mesh that shapes and nurtures skin, bones, muscles, and tendons. This portion of the experiment indicates that Zinc-Carnosine does not have a direct effect on the growth of mucosal cells in the lining of the stomach.

- Zinc-Carnosine caused an increase in the gene expression of IGF-1 in endothelial and fibroblast cells. This could provide a clue as to how Zinc-Carnosine affects cells in the stomach lining. It could be that Zinc-Carnosine makes stomach epithelial cells grow and develop by means of a paracrine action. In other words, IGF-1 produced in endothelial cells may be passed to epithelial cells on the stomach lining.

- Zinc-Carnosine dramatically increased the growth and development of endothelial and fibroblast cells. By contrast, L-carnosine alone had no effect on these cells, and zinc alone increased cell growth by a factor of two, far below the growth rate of Zinc-Carnosine. This confirmed that zinc is the essential healing component of Zinc-Carnosine, but that L-carnosine plays a very important role in the compound, because it enhances the healing power of the zinc.

Zinc-Carnosine and Prostaglandin E

In a rather ghastly but to-the-point experiment, H. Nishiwaki and his colleagues at the Kyoto Pharmaceutical University in Japan pretreated rats with 2 to 12 mg/ml of Zinc-Carnosine or 2 micrograms/ml of prostaglandin E and then had the rats swallow 1 ml of ammonia or monochloramine (the chloride of ammonia). Needless to say, these caustic substances soon caused severe hemorrhagic ulcers. However, rats pretreated with Zinc-Carnosine had smaller gastric lesions in a dose-dependent manner. Rats pretreated with prostaglandin E also had smaller lesions. The scientists then anesthetized the rats, opened their stomachs, and applied Zinc-Carnosine topically. Again, the lesions receiving higher doses of Zinc-Carnosine showed more improvement. However, this time the prostaglandin E had no effect.

This experiment is interesting because it addresses the supposition that Zinc-Carnosine is prostaglandin-independent. In other words, the supplement does not rely on prostaglandins to heal stomach tissue. As Chapter 3 explains, non-steroidal anti-inflammatory drugs (NSAIDs) interfere with prostaglandin production and, in so doing, impair the stomach's natural mucosal defenses. If Zinc-Carnosine and prostaglandins have nothing to do with each other as this experiment suggests, it is good news for ulcer patients who must take NSAIDs for their joint pain. These patients can take Zinc-Carnosine with the assurance that it will relieve pain because it doesn't rely on prostaglandins to do so.

Zinc-Carnosine's Interaction with Various Drugs

In an experiment conducted by S. Kato et al. involving Zinc-Carnosine and the stomach's mucosal layer, scientists in Kyoto Pharmaceutical University performed another ghastly experiment on rats, this one involving Zinc-Carnosine and sucralfate. As Chapter 6 explains, sucralfate (Sulcrate, Antipepsin, Carafate) is a polymer that coats the stomach to form a barrier between an ulcer and gastric acid. The drug can be purchased over-the-counter. It is not a first-line treatment for ulcers, but it is still used in treatments, especially in Japan. For the experiment, scientists pretreated rats with Zinc-Carnosine (3 to 30 mg/kg), but this time the rats were pretreated as well with significant amounts of sucralfate (30 and 100 mg/kg) and indomethacin, an anti-inflammatory drug. Then the rats were fed monochloramine (the chloride of ammonia). This caused massive lipid peroxidation—free radicals "stealing" electrons from cell membrane lipids to cause cell damage—and severe hemorrhaging.

The scientists reported that the protective effect of Zinc-Carnosine on the stomach was not affected by indomethacin, but that the protective effect of sucralfate was lessened. This experiment was interesting because much higher doses of sucralfate than Zinc-Carnosine were needed to protect the stomach, and, Zinc-Carnosine worked in spite of the presence of the anti-inflammatory indomethacin, whereas sucralfate did not work. This indicates that Zinc-Carnosine is worth considering as a treatment for peptic ulcer disease in patients who are taking indomethacin for arthritis pain and inflammation.

Apoptosis is the self-destruction, or death, of cells that normally occurs when cells become abnormal. Cancer occurs when apoptosis fails and malignant cells that normally die are permitted to keep living. On the other hand, when you age, too much apoptosis occurs. Certain genes are associated with apoptosis. When these genes are switched on, cells die. Indomethacin, a drug that doctors prescribe to arthritis patients to lower inflammation, causes apoptosis in certain types of cells.

To test the effectiveness of Zinc-Carnosine when it is used in combination with indomethacin, Y. Fuji et al. at Tottori University in Yonago, Japan, looked at the effect of Zinc-Carnosine on indomethacin-induced apoptosis in mucosal cells from rats' stomachs. The researchers discovered that Zinc-Carnosine, in amounts as low as 5 microM, inhibited cell apoptosis, and that 50 microM exhibited the maximum inhibitory effect. The scientists determined that zinc, not L-carnosine, played the primary role in inhibiting apoptosis. It appears the Zinc-Carnosine gives cells— that would otherwise die by apoptosis at the hands of an anti-inflammatory drug—an encouraging message to keep on living.

Zinc-Carnosine in Quadruple Drug Therapies for H. Pylori-Caused Ulcers

As Chapter 6 explains, the standard treatment for *H. pylori*-induced ulcers is a triple or quadruple therapy consisting of two or three antibiotics and one or two other drugs, usually a proton pump inhibitor or H_2 blocker.

A very interesting study conducted at the Jutendo School of Medicine in Tokyo threw Zinc-Carnosine into this mix. It attempted to discover if Zinc-Carnosine could be useful along with other drugs in a quadruple-therapy treatment for *H. pylori*-caused ulcers. The experiment involved two antibiotics (amoxicillin and clarithromycin), the proton pump inhibitor lansoprazole, and Zinc-Carnosine. Sixty-six ulcer patients with *H. pylori* infections and dyspepsia took part in the seven-day study. The subjects were divided into two groups. Group A, with thirty-one patients, received lansoprazole (30 mg twice a day), amoxicillin (500 mg twice a day), and clarithromycin (400 mg twice a day). Group B, with thirty-five patients, received the same regimen plus Zinc-Carnosine (75 mg twice a day). Five patients left the study due to severe diarrhea (a side effect of antibiotic treatment). Of the patients who remained, twenty-four of twenty-eight, or 86 percent, in Group A were rid of their *H. pylori* infections. In Group B, thirty-three of thirty-three, or 100 percent, of subjects were no longer infected with *II. pylori*. In this study, Zinc-Carnosine significantly improved the cure rate of *H. pylori*-induced ulcers in a seven-day quadruple-therapy regimen. By restoring the health of the mucosa, Zinc-Carnosine may improve the stomach lining's ability to fight off an *H. pylori* infection.

Dosage

So how much Zinc-Carnosine should you take? The standard adult dosage of Zinc-Carnosine is 75 mg a day—or, better still, 37.5 mg twice daily—to be taken for eight weeks. Usually, the supplement is taken in tablet form once in the morning and once before bed. It is best taken with food. The cost of using the supplement is eighty cents to one dollar per day.

Studies have shown that the optimal dose of Zinc-Carnosine is 150 mg per day, not 75 mg. However, I recommend taking 75 mg daily because, first, studies show that the effects of the optimal dose and recommended dose are actually quite similar, and, second, taking 75 instead of 150 mg per day enables patients to meet, but not exceed, the FDA's recommended daily intake (RDI) of zinc. Zinc-Carnosine has been studied on men and women in the 16- to 75-age range, but as yet, no independent studies have been conducted on children, pregnant women, or nursing mothers. Check with your healthcare practitioner before you take Zinc-Carnosine if you are in one of those groups. In any case, peptic ulcer disease is very uncommon in children.

Is It Safe?

Of course, the first question to ask about any drug or supplement is, "Is it safe?" The answer where Zinc-Carnosine is concerned is a definitive "yes." Because the supplement contains zinc, toxicity is a concern. But, as I will explain below, zinc is not really a problem. Moreover, the supplement has shown a remarkable lack of side effects. This is good news for people with peptic ulcer disease. The majority of drugs used to treat the disease—proton pump inhibitors and antibiotics—come with very uncomfortable side effects. Remember, though, that no independent safety studies have been conducted regarding the use of Zinc-Carnosine on children, pregnant women, or nursing mothers.

Toxicity Concerns

For adults, 15 mg is the recommended daily intake (RDI) of zinc. The zinc content in Zinc-Carnosine is 22 percent. The recommended dose is 75 mg daily, which means that a person taking Zinc-Carnosine gets roughly 15 mg of zinc per day. This is the same amount of zinc found in multivitamins such as One-A-Day. Moreover, this is well below the 40 mg tolerable upper limit (TUI) established by the National Academy of Sciences for adults. Even a person taking Zinc-Carnosine along with a daily multivitamin will not exceed the TUI for zinc.

Copper deficiency is a concern to anyone taking zinc supplements because high doses of zinc retard the body's ability to absorb copper. Copper is needed for producing red blood cells and manufacturing insulin. It also plays a role in iron absorption. Still, someone would have to take an enormous amount of Zinc-Carnosine to be deficient in copper. People taking a multivitamin and Zinc-Carnosine are unlikely to acquire a copper deficiency, because multivitamins contain copper.

For safety purposes, the Zeria Pharmaceutical Company in Japan conducted two studies on zinc and copper as they pertain to the consumption of Zinc-Carnosine:

- Scientists examined zinc and copper residues in the blood and organs of rats that received repeated doses of Zinc-Carnosine. In animals that received 75 mg/kg—more than 60 times the dosage in humans!—for fifty-two weeks, no toxicity was observed. Tissue zinc and copper concentrations were unaffected. At doses of 150 mg/kg for fifty-two weeks, the rats' zinc levels showed a slight increase in the blood, liver, and kidneys, but the copper levels were not affected. Animals given 300 mg/kg—the equivalent of a human being taking two hundred Zinc-Carnosine capsules a day—for a year experienced decreased copper levels in their blood, liver, kidneys, testes, lungs, and spleen. After five weeks of withdrawal from Zinc-Carnosine, however, the rats' zinc and copper levels returned to normal.

- Using radioactive tracers, scientists found that zinc levels in the blood returned to their previous levels eleven hours after taking Zinc-Carnosine; zinc concentrations in the liver, kidneys, testicles, prostate gland, and brain remained constant. The zinc in Zinc-Carnosine did not cross the blood-testis or blood-brain barrier.

A 75-mg daily dose of Zinc-Carnosine provides about 60 mg per day of L-carnosine. This is nowhere near the 400 to 500 mg of L-carnosine found, for example, in a quarter pound of pork. The L-carnosine in Zinc-Carnosine is harmless.

Toxicity expert Dr. Robert A. DiSilvestro—in a review of studies relevant to the safety of Zinc-Carnosine submitted to the FDA as part of the supplement's new dietary ingredient review—had this to say about Zinc-Carnosine's safety: "At present, I can see no reason to expect toxicity from a daily dose of 75 mg of Z-103 (Zinc-Carnosine). The two individual constituents of Z-103 are already normal components of the human body, the amounts administered are not large compared to other ways of ingesting these constituents, and current research in vitro, in animals, and in humans all give evidence of safety."

Side Effects and Adverse Effects

In a meta-analysis of studies done on Zinc-Carnosine, Dr. Bernd

Wollschlaeger found no adverse effects from the supplement. One double-blind study reported a subject with nausea and one with numbness in the lips, and another study reported a case of edema, but these side effects could well have been caused by something besides Zinc-Carnosine. None of the patients with side effects required further evaluation or treatment.

Disadvantages

I should pause a moment and explain the supplement's disadvantages. As I see it, there is only one drawback: As with most natural products, Zinc-Carnosine does not stop ulcer pain right away, in the same manner as a proton pump inhibitor. Pain relief is gradual, with most people feeling some relief after two weeks, and substantial relief at the end of the eight-week course of treatment. Needless to say, immediate relief from pain is a powerful incentive to keep taking a drug or supplement. People who take Zinc-Carnosine don't have this incentive. However, Zinc-Carnosine offers long-lasting relief from ulcer pain because it treats the disease's causes as well as its symptoms. Most drug treatments, by contrast, address only symptoms. For example, they suppress acid production in the stomach, but do nothing to address the ulcer sore that caused the pain to begin with.

CONCLUSION

Now that you know a little more about Zinc-Carnosine, make sure you don't use it as a substitute for medical advice. As excited as I am about this supplement, I must urge you to seek evaluation by a healthcare professional. If it is determined that your problem is a peptic ulcer, then by all means, ask your physician about Zinc-Carnosine. If your doctor is not familiar with the supplement, feel free to bring in this book. As my father used to say, "You're never too old to learn."

Conclusion

I hope you found this book both informative and empowering. With the "normal" stresses in our daily existence, our woefully inadequate modern-day diets, and the less-than-friendly environment in which we sometimes find ourselves, it's no wonder so many of us suffer from a host of stomach ailments. By writing this book, I have tried to provide the individual looking for relief a balanced view of effective peptic ulcer disease treatments—covering conventional, alternative, and breakthrough therapies.

There are, however, a few things I'd like to mention in closing. One is the overuse of antacids in this country. When we become accustomed to consuming antacids like candies without any regard to their accumulative effects on our body, we only add to our health problems. Antacid tablets are a Catch-22, in that they relieve ulcer pain but also hide pain and permit ulcers to remain—without being treated. H_2-blocking drugs were originally prescription drugs, but now they are sold over-the-counter, and, not surprisingly, some people pop these inexpensive pills without any regard for the long-term health consequences. H_2 blockers, and proton pump inhibitors as well, interfere with the metabolism of the stomach. They lower stomach acidity, which relieves ulcer pain, but they also permit germs and pathogens that would otherwise be killed by acid to survive. Moreover, they interfere with the absorption of protein and vitamin B_{12}. Remember that the digestive tract is a continuum, and that disrupting it in one area always has health consequences further down the line.

One final word: If, after reading this book, you do nothing to alleviate your condition, then—in fact—you are a victim of your own choosing. This book was designed to offer you a wide range of ways to treat and cure your problem. If you are afraid of visiting your doctor because of what he or she may find, remember that the odds are good that your condition is very treatable. Waiting until the condition worsens can only complicate matters. Forty years ago, it took an order from an Army doctor for me to go for help. If that's what it takes, consider this book your marching orders.

Glossary

achlorhydria: The prolonged absence of gastric acid secretion in the stomach.

acid rebound: The increase of gastric acid, as, for example, when acid secretion is stimulated by the calcium carbonate in antacids.

air-contrast upper GI: *See* double-contrast radiography.

antacid: An alkaline designed to neutralize hydrochloric acid (HCl) in the stomach and relieve gastric pain.

antrectomy: Surgical removal of the antrum, or lower half of the stomach. Most stomach acid is produced and most stomach ulcers occur in the antrum. Removing this portion of the stomach lowers acid production and leaves a smaller stomach area for ulcers to form.

antrum: The lower area of the stomach immediately before the small intestine.

barium swallow: An examination of the pharynx and esophagus by radiography. *See also* radiography.

barium: A low-grade radioactive metallic liquid used to make the interior surfaces of the body visible in radiography X-rays. *See also* radiography.

basal acid output (BAO): The amount of gastric acid secreted in the stomach in the absence of stimulation.

bicarbonates: Alkaline substances (in the stomach) that neutralize gastric acid and help protect the stomach from damage. Some bicarbonates are produced by the pancreas.

biopsy: Removal of tissue from patients for diagnostic examination. Also, the tissue removed by biopsy.

borborygmi: Rumbling noises from the gastrointestinal tract.

diverticulum: A pouch or a pocket-like opening in the wall of the bowel.

double-contrast radiography: In a radiology examination, when patients swallow baking-soda crystals as well as barium. The crystals create gas and help to improve X-ray images. *See also* radiography.

duodenal bulb: The first part of the duodenum that connects the duodenum to the stomach. This is also called the duodenal cap. *See also* duodenum.

duodenal ulcer: An ulcer that occurs in the duodenum, the first portion of the small intestine. *See also* peptic ulcer.

duodenum: The first portion of the small intestine, about ten inches long. It conveys the same acidic environment as the stomach.

dyspepsia: A persistent or recurring pain or discomfort located in the upper abdomen.

endoscope: A flexible fiberoptic instrument through which doctors can examine and take biopsies from the esophagus, stomach, duodenum, and other organs.

endoscopy: The examination of a patient by means of an endoscope. This is also called a gastroscopy when examining the stomach. *See also* endoscope.

epigastrium: The upper middle third of the abdomen, directly below the diaphragm.

esophagitis: Inflammation of the walls of the esophagus.

esophagus: The muscular tube-like structure, approximately nine inches long, that connects the throat to the stomach. This is also called the gullet.

fistula: An abnormal opening, or tunnel, between one organ and another or the surface of the skin.

fundus: The convex upper portion, or roof, of the stomach.

gastric acid: A general term for hydrochloric acid, pepsinogen, and other substances secreted by the epithelial glands for the purpose of breaking down food in the stomach. *See also* hydrochloric acid (HCl).

gastric adaptation: The process whereby the stomach heals on its own from gastric erosions caused by taking NSAIDs.

gastric ulcer: An ulcer that occurs in the stomach. *See also* duodenal ulcer and peptic ulcer.

gastrin: A hormone that regulates the production of hydrochloric acid (HCl) in the stomach.

gastrinoma: A malignant, gastrin-secreting tumor that causes excessive production of hydrochloric acid (HCl) in the stomach, and, consequently, tumors in the stomach and duodenum.

gastritis: Chronic inflammation of the stomach lining.

gastroenterostomy: A procedure in which the stomach is surgically connected to the small intestine, usually the jejunum, the middle portion of the small intestine.

gastroesophageal reflux disease (GERD): A condition in which acid from the stomach persistently rises into the esophagus to cause discomfort and heartburn.

gastrointestinal tract: The parts of the body, from the salivary glands to the anus, that are responsible for absorbing or expelling food.

gastroscope: An endoscope designed for examining the esophagus, stomach, and duodenum. *See also* endoscope.

gastroscopy: An endoscopy performed on the stomach and duodenum. *See also* endoscopy.

gastrostomy: The establishment of a new opening into the stomach.

g-cells: Cells in the stomach that produce gastrin, a hormone involved in parietal cells' production of hydrochloric acid.

GERD: *See* gastroesophageal reflux disease.

GI tract: *See* gastrointestinal tract.

gullet: *See* esophagus.

H. pylori: See Helicobacter pylori.

H₂-blocking drug: A drug that affects parietal cells in the stomach to inhibit the production of hydrochloric acid and relieve heartburn and indigestion. Also called H₂ receptor antagonists and H₂ blockers.

HCl: *See* hydrochloric acid.

Helicobacter pylori (H. pylori): The bacterium that can causes gastritis, stomach ulcers, and ulcers of the duodenum. The genus name (*Helicobacter*) refers to the bacterium's helical, or spiral, shape; the species name (*pylori*) refers to the pyloric valve, the sphincter muscle that separates the stomach from the duodenum.

hematemesis: The presence of blood in vomit.

hematochezia: The medical term for passing stools that are red or maroon-colored due to bleeding in the large intestine or rectum. *See also* melena.

hydrochloric acid (HCl): Acid produced in the stomach to break down food and kill bacteria and other germs.

jejunum: The second portion of the small intestine, about eight feet long, where nutrients from food are absorbed and passed through to the bloodstream.

melena: Medical term for passing stools that are black, tarry, and foul-smelling on account of severe bleeding in the upper gastrointestinal tract. *See also* hematochezia.

non-steroidal anti-inflammatory drugs: *See* NSAIDs.

NSAIDs: Acronym for non-steroidal anti-inflammatory drugs, the pain-relieving and anti-inflammatory drug category that includes aspirin and ibuprofen. Pronounced "EN-seds."

oesophagus: The British spelling of esophagus.

over-the-counter: A term which describes drugs that are available without a prescription.

parietal cells: Cells in the stomach that secrete hydrochloric acid (HCl).

pepsin: An enzyme produced in the mucosal lining of the stomach that begins to break down dietary proteins into peptides and amino acids so that they can be absorbed in the small intestine.

peptic ulcer: The general term for gastric (stomach) and duodenal ulcers. "Peptic" refers to a part of the body where digestion takes place and acid is present.

perforation: The condition in which an ulcer sore penetrates the wall of the stomach or duodenum, and gastric acid and other stomach contents leak into the peritoneum to cause an inflammation or infection in the form of peritonitis.

peritoneum: The membrane that lines the wall of the abdomen and covers the abdominal organs.

pharynx: The part of the throat, from behind the nose to the beginning of the voice box, that is a common pathway for food and air.

prostaglandins: Hormone-like substances that regulate pain messaging, mucus production in the stomach, and other body functions. NSAIDs work by inhibiting the production of prostaglandins.

proton pump inhibitor (PPI): A drug that blocks the action of the proton pump in the stomach's parietal cells and, in so doing, decreases or stops the production of hydrochloric acid.

proton pump: The enzyme system responsible for releasing hydrochloric acid from parietal cells in the stomach. The biochemical name is hydrogen-potassium adenosine triphosphatase (H + ,K + -ATPase).

radiography: A means of X-raying a part of the body for diagnostic purposes.

single-contrast radiography: *See* double-contrast radiography.

small intestine: The upper portion of the intestine, comprising the duodenum, jejunum, and ileum.

string test: A means of obtaining gastric juice for *H. pylori* evaluation. For the test, subjects swallow a string that is later retrieved for analysis.

ulcer: A deep lesion or crater sore on the mucosa or lining of the stomach or duodenal wall that is surrounded by acute inflammation.

ulcerative colitis: The ulceration of the colon and rectum, character-ized by abdominal pain and rectal bleeding.

upper gastrointestinal (GI) series: A radiography test that provides a series of video-like X-ray images of the esophagus, stomach, and duodenum. This is also called an upper GI series. *See also* radiography.

vagotomy: Surgical cutting of the vagus nerve to reduce the secretion of hydrochloric acid in the stomach.

vagus nerve: The nerve by which the signal to produce gastrin is passed from the brain to the parietal cells of the stomach. *See also* gas-trin.

References

Chapter 1

Bartle WR et al (1986) Nonsteroidal anti-inflammatory drugs and gastrointestinal bleeding: A case-control study. *Arch Intern Med* 146:2365.

Bloom BS (1991) Cross-national changes in the effects of peptic ulcer disease. *Ann Intern Med* 114:558.

Graham DY (1989) Complications of peptic ulcer disease and indications for surgery. In Sleisenger et al eds, *Gastrointestinal Disease: Pathophysiology, Diagnosis, Management.* Philadelphia, PA: WB Saunders.

Henry D et al (1993) Nonsteroidal anti-inflammatory drugs and peptic ulcer hospitalization rates in New South Wales. *Gastroenterology.* 104:1083.

Kurata JH (1991) Epidemiology of peptic ulcer disease. In Swabb EA et al eds. *Ulcer Disease: Investigation and Basis for Therapy.* New York, NY: Marcel Dekker; 31.

Rogers AI (1997) Peptic ulcer disease: Retracing science's journey through the gut. *Postgrad Med* 102;5:158.

Smalley WE et al (1996) The risks and costs of upper gastrointestinal disease attributable to NSAIDs. *Gastroenterol Clin North Am* 25:373–396.

Sonnenberg A et al (1997) Health impact of peptic ulcer in the United States. *Am J Gastroenterol* 92(4):614–620.

Thompson WG (1996) *The Ulcer Story.* New York, NY: Plenum Publishing Corp; 3-26, 33–58.

Chapter 2

Andermann TM et al (2002) Two predicted chemoreceptors promote *Helicobacter pylori* infection. *Infection Immunity* 70:5877–5881.

Argyros F et al (2000) Evaluation of a PCR primer based on the isocitrate dehydrogenase gene for detection of *Helicobacter pylori* in feces. *J Clin Microbiol* 38:10; 3755–3758.

Blaser MJ (1996) The bacteria behind ulcers. *Scientific American.* 274:2;104–107.

Blaser MJ (1997) Not all *Helicobacter pylori* strains are created equal; should all be eliminated? *Lancet* 349:1020–22.

Blaser MJ (1999) In a world of black and white, *Helicobacter pylori* is gray. *Ann Intern Med* 130;8:695–697.

Boren T et al (1998) *Helicobacter pylori* adhesin binding fucosylated histo-blood group antigens revealed by retagging. *Science* 279(5349):373–7.

Chey WD et al (1999) The ^{13}C-urea blood test accurately detects active *Helicobacter pylori* infection: A United States, multicenter trial. *Am J Gastroenterol* 94:1522–1524.

Chow WH et al (1998) An inverse relation between *cagA*+ strains of *Helicobacter pylori* infection and risk of esophageal and gastric cardia adeno-carcinoma. *Cancer Res* 58:588–590.

Cullen DJ (1993) When is *Helicobacter pylori* infection acquired? *Gut* 34:1681–1682.

Currey R (1998) Barry Marshall: Persistence paid off. *Snapshots of medicine and science.* Oct 15. http://science-education.nih.gov/Snapshots.nsf/story?openForm&rtn~SB_Hpylori_Marshall

Eurogast Study Group (1993). International gastric cancer rates correlate with rates of HP seropositivity. *Lancet* 341(8857):1359–361.

Goodwin CS et al (1993) The *Helicobacter* genus: The history of *H. pylori* and taxonomy of current species. In Goodwin CS et al (Eds), *Helicobacter pylori: Biology and clinical practice.* Boca Raton: CRC Press. 1–13.

Graham DY (1993). Treatment of peptic ulcers caused by *Helicobacter pylori. N Engl J Med* 328; 349–350.

Graham DY (1997). Can therapy even be denied for *Helicobacter pylori* infection? *Gastroenterology* 113(6 Suppl):S113–7

Graham DY et al (1991) Epidemiology of *Helicobacter pylori* in an asymptomatic population in the United States: Effect of age, race, and socio-economic status. *Gastroenterology* 100(6):1495–501.

Graham DY et al (1998) *H pylori* and *cagA:* Relationships with gastric cancer, duodenal ulcer, and reflux esophagitis and its complications. *Helicobacter* 3(3):145–51.

Graham S (2002) Stomach sugars could be key to ulcer vaccine. *Scientific American.com* July 26. http://www.sciam.com/article.cfm?articleID= 000E74D5-5ECF-1D40-90FB809EC5880000.

Howden CW et al (1998) Guidelines for the management of *Helicobacter pylori* infection. *Am J Gastroenterol* 93(12):2330–2338.

Hulten K et al (1996) *Helicobacter pylori* in the drinking water in Peru. *Gastroenterology* 110(4):1031–5.

Jones AD et al (2003) *Helicobacter pylori* induces apoptosis in Barrett's-derived esophageal adenocarcinoma cells. *J Gastrointest Surg* 7(1):68–76.

Kalayoglu MV et al (2002) *Chlamydia pneumoniae* as an emerging risk factor in cardiovascular disease. *JAMA* 4;288(21):2724–31.

Kaptan K (2000). *Helicobacter pylori*—Is it a novel causative agent in vitamin B_{12} deficiency? *Arch Intern Med* 60:1349–1353.

Kerr JR et al (2000) An association between sudden infant death syndrome (SIDS) and *Helicobacter pylori* infection. *Arch Dis Child* 83(5): 429–34.

Labenz J et al (1997) Curing *Helicobacter pylori* infection in patients with duodenal ulcer may provoke reflux esophagitis. *Gastroenterology* 112:1442–7.

Lin SK et al (1991) Comparison of *Helicobacter pylori* in three ethnic groups evidence for oral-oral transmission. *Gastroenterology* 100;5(2): A111.

Malaty HM et al (2002) Age at acquisition of *Helicobacter pylori* infection: A follow-up study from infancy to adulthood. *Lancet* 359:931–5.

Marshall BJ et al (1983) Unidentified curved bacilli on gastric epithelium in active chronic gastritis. *Lancet* 1:1273–5.

Marshall BJ et al (1988) Prospective double-blind trial of duodenal ulcer relapse after eradication of *Campylobacter pylori*. *Lancet* 2(8626/8627); 1437–1441.

Martensen R (1994) Cancer: Medical history and the framing of a disease. *JAMA* 271:24–28.

McDonnell P (2002) Stomach-dwelling *H. pylori* bacterium reveals its age. New York University Medical Center and School of Medicine press release. November 4. http://www.eurekalert.org/pub_releases/2002-11/nyum-shp103102.php

Mitchell HM et al (1992) Epidemiology of *Helicobacter pylori* in southern China: Identification of early childhood as the critical period for acquisition. *J Infect Dis* 166(1):149–53.

Monmaney T (1993) Marshall's hunch. *New Yorker*, September 20; 64–72.

Newcombe R (2003) Could there be an obesity virus? *BUPA investigative news* 10 January http://www.bupa.co.uk/health_information/html/health_news/100103fatvirus.html

NIH Consensus Conference (1994) *Helicobacter pylori* in peptic ulcer disease: NIH Consensus Development Panel on *Helicobacter pylori* in peptic ulcer disease. *JAMA* 272:65–9.

Ottemann KM et al (2002) *Helicobacter pylori* uses motility for initial colonization and to attain robust infection. *Infection Immunity* 70:1984–1990.

Peek RM et al (1997) Pathophysiology of *Helicobacter pylori*-induced gastritis and peptic ulcer disease. *Am J Med* 102(2): 200–7.

Salama N et al (2000) A whole-genome microarray reveals diversity among *Helicobacter pylori* strains. *PNAS* 97(26):14668–14673.

Susser M (1982) Period effects, generation effects and age effects in peptic ulcer mortality. *J Chronic Dis* 35:29.

Suzuki D (1995). Ulcer wars. *The Nature of Things* (originally produced by BBC TV).

Thompson WG (1996) *The Ulcer Story.* New York, NY: Plenum Publishing Corp; 93–104.

Touchette N (2003) *H. pylori* paradox: Microbe harms stomach but protects esophagus. *Genome News Network* http://www.genomenewsnetwork.org/ articles/04_03/pylori.shtml.

U.S. Department of Health and Human Services, public Health Service, National Institutes of Health (1994) *Digestive diseases in the United States: Epidemiology and impact.* Publication 94–1447. Washington, DC.

Walboomers JM et al (1999) Human papillomavirus is a necessary cause of invasive cervical cancer worldwide. *J Pathol* 189(1):12–19.

Chapter 3

Akil M et al (1996) Infertility may sometimes be associated with NSAID consumption. *Br J Rheumatol* 35;1:76–8.

Armstrong CP et al (1987) Non-steroidal anti-inflammatory drugs and life-threatening complications of peptic ulceration. *Gut* 28:527–532.

Bas A. et al (2001) Nonsteroidal antiinflammatory drugs and the risk of Alzheimer's disease *N Engl J Med* 21;345:1515–1521.

Brater DC et al (2001) Renal effects of COX-2-selective inhibitors. *Am J Nephrol* 21(1):1–15

Brennan MR (2003) The cost-effectiveness of cyclooxygenase-2 selective inhibitors in the management of chronic arthritis. *Ann Intern Med* 138; 10:795–806.

Brown D (2001) Heart risk from Celebrex, Vioxx? *Washington Post* August 22:A04.

Chandrasekharan NV et al (2002) COX-3, a cyclooxygenase-1 variant inhibited by acetaminophen and other analgesic/antipyretic drugs: Cloning, structure, and expression. *Proc Natl Acad Sci USA* 99(21):13926–31.

Conn HO (1994) Corticosteroids and peptic ulcer: Meta-analysis of adverse events during steroid therapy. *J Int Med* 236(6):619–32.

Conn HO et al (1976) Nonassociation of adrenocorticosteroid therapy and peptic ulcer. *N Eng J Med* 294:73.

De-Kun Li et al (2003) Exposure to non-steroidal anti-inflammatory drugs during pregnancy and risk of miscarriage: Population based cohort study *BMJ* 327:368.

Diabetic News (2002) Evidence shows aspirin reduces risk of a first heart attack. Nov 18. http://diabeticgourmet.com/tdn/news/421.shtml.

Goggin PM et al (1993) Prevalence of *Helicobacter pylori* infection and its effect or symptoms and non-steroidal anti-inflammatory drug induced gastrointestinal damage in patients with rheumatoid arthritis. *Gut* 34:1677–1680.

Goldstein JL (1998) Public misunderstanding of nonsteroidal antiinflammatory drug (NSAID)-mediated gastrointestinal complications toxicity: A serious potential health threat. *Gastroenterology* 114:G0555.

Graham DY (1988) Prevention of NSAID-induced gastric ulcer with misoprostol: Multicentre, double-blind, placebo-controlled trial. *Lancet* 2(8623):1277–1280.

Messer J et al (1983) Association of adrenocorticosteroid therapy and peptic-ulcer disease. *N Eng J Med* 309:21.

Graham DY et al (1986) Aspirin and the stomach. *Ann Intern Med* 104(3):390–398.

Graham DY et al (1991) Long-term non-steroidal anti-inflammatory drug use and *Helicobacter pylori* infection. *Gastroenterology* 100:1653.

Graumlich JF (2001) Preventing gastrointestinal complications of NSAIDs: Risk factors, recent advances, and latest strategies. *Postgrad Med* 109(5):117–128.

Griffin MR et al (1991). Nonsteroidal anti-inflammatory drug use and death from peptic ulcer in elderly persons. *Ann Intern Med* 114:257.

Gunnar Lauge Nielsen et al (2001) Risk of adverse birth outcome and miscarriage in pregnant users of non-steroidal anti-inflammatory drugs: Population based observational study and case-control study. *BMJ* 322:266–270.

Hernandez-Diaz S et al (2000) Association between nonsteroidal anti-inflammatory drugs and upper gastrointestinal tract bleeding/perforation: An overview of epidemiologic studies published in the 1990s. *Arch Intern Med* 160(14):2093–2099.

Ivey KJ (1988) Mechanisms of nonsteroidal anti-inflammatory drug-induced gastric damage; actions of therapeutic agents. *Am J Med* 88:41.

Jane VR (1971) Inhibition of prostaglandin synthesis as a mechanism of action for aspirin-like drugs. *Nat N Biol* 231:232–235.

Kurata J et al (1990) The effect of chronic aspirin use on duodenal and gastric ulcer hospitalization. *J Clin Gastroenterol* 12:260.

La Corte R et al (1999) Prophylaxis and treatment of NSAID-induced gastroduodenal disorders. *Drug Saf* 20(6):527–543.

Li EKM et al (1996) *Helicobacter pylori* infection increases the risk of peptic ulcers in chronic users of non-steroidal anti-inflammatory drugs. *Scand J Rheumatol* 25:42–46.

Lieberman T (2001) When hype stands in for solid science. *Los Angeles Times* June 18.

Mukherjee D et al (2001) Risk of cardiovascular events associated with selective COX-2 inhibitors. *JAMA* 286:954–959.

Primack WA et al (1997) Acute renal failure associated with amoxicillin and ibuprofen in an 11-year-old boy. *Pediatr Nephrol* 11:125–126.

Publig W et al (1994) Non-steroidal anti-inflammatory drugs (NSAIDs) cause gastrointestinal ulcers mainly in *Helicobacter pylori* carriers. *Wien Klin Wochenschr* 106: 276–279.

Redfern JS et al (1989) Role of endogenous prostaglandins in preventing gastrointestinal ulceration: Induction of ulcers by anti-bodies to prostaglandins. *Gastroenterology* 96:596.

Riley TR et al (1998) Ibuprofen-induced hepatotoxicity in patients with chronic hepatitis C: A case series. *Am J Gastroenterol* 93(9):1563–1565.

Sandler RS (1998) Aspirin and nonsteroidal anti-inflammatory agents and risk for colorectal adenomas *Gastroenterology* 114:441–7.

Schoen RT et al (1989) Mechanisms of nonsteroidal anti-inflammatory drug-induced gastric damage. *Am J Med* 86:449.

Singh G (1996) Gastrointestinal tract complications of nonsteroidal anti-inflamatory drug treatment in rheumatoid arthritis. *Arch Intern Med* 156:1530–1536.

Smith G et al (1996) Reversible ovulatory failure associated with the development of luteinized unruptured follicles in women with inflammatory arthritis taking non-steroidal anti-inflammatory drugs. *Br J Rheum* 35: 5, 458–62.

Steering Committee of the Physicians' Health Study Research Group. Final report on the aspirin component of the ongoing Physicians' Health Study. *N Eng J Med* 321:129–135.

Steinbach G. et al (2000) The effect of celecoxib, a cyclooxygenase-2 inhibitor, in familial adenomatous polyposis. *N Engl J Med* 342:1946–1952.

Stone E (1763) An account of the success of the bark of the willow in the cure of agues. *Philos Trans* 53:195–200.

Swan SK et al (2000) Effect of cyclooxygenase-2 inhibition on renal function in elderly persons receiving a low-salt diet. *Ann Intern Med* 133:1–9.

Thompson WG (1996) *The Ulcer Story.* New York, NY: Plenum Publishing Corp; 81–92.

Warner TD et al (2002) Cyclooxygenase-3 (COX-3): Filling in the gaps toward a COX continuum? *Proc Natl Acad Sci USA* 99(21):13371–13373.

Weggen S et al (2001) A subset of NSAIDs lower amyloidogenic AB42 independently of cyclooxygenase activity. *Nature* 414:212–216.

Wolfe M et al (1999) Gastrointestinal toxicity of nonsteroidal anti-inflammatory drugs. *N Engl J Med* 340;24:1888–1889.

Chapter 4

Adami HO (1987) Is duodenal ulcer really a psychosomatic disease? A population-based case-control study. *Scand J Gastroenterol* 22:889.

Ainsworth MA et al (1993) Cigarette smoking inhibits acid-stimulated duodenal mucosal bicarbonate secretion. *Ann Intern Med* 119:882–886.

Arakawa T et al (2000) *Helicobacter pylori:* Criminal or innocent bystander? *J Gastroenterol* 35(Suppl-12):42–46.

Baena J et al (2002) Relation between alcohol consumption and the success of *Helicobacter pylori* eradication therapy using omeprazole, clarithromycin and amoxicillin for 1 week. *Eur J Gastroenterol Hepatol* 14;3:291–296.

Bresalier R (1991) The clinical significance and pathophysiology of stress-related gastric mucosal hemorrhage. *J Clin Gastroenterol* 13(Suppl 2):S35.

Carey J (1992) What Barry Marshall knew in his gut. *Business Week* 10:68–69.

Chan FK et al (1997) Does smoking predispose to peptic ulcer relapse after eradication of *Helicobacter pylori*? *Am J Gastroenterol* 92(3):442–445.

Cohen S et al (1975) Gastric acid secretion and lower-esophageal-sphincter pressure in response to coffee and caffeine. *N Engl J Med* 293:897–899.

Cook D et al (1994) Risk factors for gastrointestinal bleeding in critically ill patients. *N Engl J Med* 330:377.

Elmståhl S et al (1998) Fermented milk products are associated to ulcer disease; Results from a cross-sectional population study. *Eur J Clin Nutr* 52:9;668–674.

Flynn WE (1970) Managing the emotional aspects of peptic ulcer and ulcerative colitis. *Postgrad Med* 47(5):119–22.

Graham DY (1993) Treatment of peptic ulcers caused by *Helicobacter pylori*. *N Eng J Med*. 328(5):349–350.

Hein HO et al (1997) Genetic markers for peptic ulcer. A study of 3387 men aged 54 to 74 years: The Copenhagen male study. *Scand J Gastroenterol* 32(1):16–21.

Hoda M et al (1994) *Helicobacter pylori* infection. Genetic and environmental influences: A study of twins. *Ann Intern Med* 120;12:982–986.

Jyotheeswaran S et al (1998) Prevalence of *Helicobacter pylori* in peptic ulcer patients in greater Rochester, NY: Is empirical triple therapy justified? *Amer J Gastroenterology* 93:574–578.

Murray LJ et al (2002) Inverse relationship between alcohol consumption and active *Helicobacter pylori* infection: Bristol Helicobacter Project. *Amer J Gastroenterol* 97:2750–2755.

Odeigah PG (1990) Influence of blood group and secretor genes on susceptibility to duodenal ulcer. *East Afr Med J* 67:487–500.

Ostensen H et al (1985) Smoking, alcohol, coffee, and familial factors: Any associations with peptic ulcer disease? A clinically and radiologically prospective study. *Scand J Gastroenterol* 20(10):1227–1235.

Parasher G et al (2000) Smoking and peptic ulcer in the *Helicobacter pylori* era. *Eur J Gastroenterol Hepatol*. 12(8):843–853.

Rotter JI (1979) Duodenal-ulcer disease associated with elevated serum pepsinogen I: An inherited autosomal dominant disorder. *N Eng J Med*. 300:63–66.

Singer MV et al (1987) Action of ethanol and some alcoholic beverages on gastric acid secretion and release of gastrin in humans. *Gastroenterology* 93:1247.

Spiro HM (1983) *Clinical Gastroenterology,* 3rd ed., New York, NY: Macmillan Publishing Co.

Sprung DJ et al (1996) The prevalence of *Helicobacter pylori* in duodenal ulcer disease: A community-based study. *Amer J Gastroenterology* 91:1926(A169).

Susser M (1967) Causes of peptic ulcer: A selective epidemiological review. *J Chron Diseases* 20:435–456.

Tally NJ et al (1988) Suppression of emotions in essential dyspepsia and chronic duodenal ulcer: A case-control study. *Scand J Gastroenterol* 23:337.

Thomas R (1907) *The Eclectic Practice of Medicine.* Cincinnati, OH: Scudder Brothers Co; http://www.ibiblio.org/herbmed/eclectic/thomas/gastric-ulc.html.

Thompson WG (1996) *The Ulcer Story.* New York, NY: Plenum Publishing Corp; 105–112, 141–142.

US Department of Health and Human Services (1988) The health consequences of smoking. nicotine addiction. A report of the surgeon general. Rockville, Maryland: US Department of Health and Human Services, Public Health Service, Centers for Disease Control, Center for Health Promotion and Education, Office on Smoking and Health. DHHS Publication No (CDC) 88-8406.

Chapter 5

Bathe OF et al (1996) Validation of a new saliva test for *Helicobacter pylori* infection. *Can J Gastroenterol* 10;2:93–96.

Brown P et al (1978) The endoscopic, radiological, and surgical findings in chronic duodenal ulceration. *Scand J Gastroenterol* 13:557.

Christie JM et al (1996) Is saliva serology useful for the diagnosis of *Helicobacter pylori*? *Gut* 39:27–30.

Cohen H et al (1996) Evaluation of a rapid test to detect IgG antibodies to *Helicobacter pylori* using fingerstick whole blood samples. *Gastroenterol* 110:A83.

Farini R (1983) Evidence of gastric carcinoma during follow up of apparently benign gastric ulcer. *Gut* 24:A486.

Gledhill T (1987) Epidemic hypochlorhydria. *BMJ* 92:1575.

Graham DY (1989) Complications of peptic ulcer disease and indications for surgery. In Sleisenger MH et al eds, *Gastrointestinal Disease: Pathophysiology, Diagnosis, Management*. Philadelphia, PA: WB Sanders.

Hirschowitz BI (1993). Development and application of endoscopy. *Gastroenterol* 104:337–342.

Howden CW et al (1998) Guidelines for the management of *Helicobacter pylori* infection. *Am J Gastroenterol* 93(12):2330–2338.

Johnsen R et al (1991) Prevalences of endoscopic and histological findings in subjects with and without dyspepsia. *BMJ* 302:749.

Lai KC et al (1996) Bleeding ulcers have high false-negative rates for antral *Helicobacter pylori* when tested with urease test. *Gastroenterol* 110:A167.

Laufer I (1976) Assessment of the accuracy of double-contrast gastroduodenal radiology. *Gastroenterol* 71:874.

Lehmann F et al (1999) Comparison of stool immunoassay with standard methods for detecting *Helicobacter pylori* infection. *Brit Med J* 319(7222): 1409.

Leong RW (2003) Evaluation of the string test for the detection of *Helicobacter pylori*. *World J Gastroenterol* 9(2):309–311.

Loy CT et al (1996) Do commercial serological kits for *Helicobacter pylori* infection differ in accuracy? A meta-analysis. *Am J Gastroenterol* 91:1138.

Molyneux AJ (1993) *Helicobacter pylori* in gastric biopsies—should you trust the pathology report? *J R Coll Physicians Lond* 27:119.

Ramsey EJ (1979) Epidemic gastritis with hypochlorhydria. *Gastroenterol* 76:1449.

Sadowski D et al (1996) Evaluation of the Flexsure HP finger-prick blood test for detection of *Helicobacter pylori* infection. *Gastroenterol* 110:A246.

Samuels AL et al (2000) Culture of *Helicobacter pylori* from a gastric string may be an alternative to endoscopic biopsy. *J Clin Microbiol* 38:2438–2439.

Soll AH (1989) Duodenal ulcer and drug therapy. In Sleisenger MH et al eds, *Gastrointestinal Disease: Pathophysiology, Diagnosis, Management*. Phila-181delphia, PA: WB Sanders.

Talley NJ (1988) Nonulcer dyspepsia: Potential causes and pathophysiology. *Ann Intern Med* 108:865.

Talley NJ et al (1991) Functional dyspepsia: A classification with guidelines for diagnosis and management. *Gastroenterol Int* 4:145.

Thagard P (1997) Ulcers and bacteria II: Instruments, experiments, and social interactions. http://cogsci.uwaterloo.ca/Articles/Pages/Ulcers. two.html.

Thomas JE et al (1992) Isolation of *Helicobacter pylori* from human faeces. *Lancet* 340: 11941195.

Thompson WG (1996) *The Ulcer Story.* New York, NY: Plenum Publishing Corp; 153–168, 349–358.

Wang SW et al (2003) The clinical utility of string-PCR test in diagnosing *Helicobacter pylori* infection. *Hepatogastroenterol* 50(53):1208–1213.

Chapter 6

Banergee S et al (1996) Sucralfate suppresses *Helicobacter pylori* infection and reduces acid secretion by 50% in patients with duodenal ulcer. *Gastroenterology* 110:717–724.

Carlsson E et al (1986) Pharmacology and toxicology of omeprazole—with special reference to the effects on the gastric mucosa. *Scand J Gastroenterol* 21[Suppl 118]:31.

Feldman M et al (1990) Histamine$_2$-receptor antagonist . Standard therapy for acid-peptic disease (part 2). *N Eng J Med* 323:1749.

Freston JW (1997) Long-term acid control and proton pump inhibitors: Interactions and safety issues in perspective. *Am J Gastroenterol* 92(4 Suppl):51S–54S.

Gasbarrini G et al (1990) Antacids in gastric ulcer treatment: Evidence of cytoprotection. *Scand J Gastrointerol Suppl* 174:44.

Gorbach SL (1990) Bismuth therapy in gastrointestinal diseases. *Gastroenterology* 99:863.

Graham DY et al (1993) Duodenal and gastric ulcer prevention with misoprostol in arthritis patients taking NSAIDs. *Ann Intern Med* 119:257–262.

Howdon CW (1991) Clinical pharmacology of omeprazole. *Clin Pharmacokinet* 20:38.

Karim QN et al (1996) Emerging patterns of *Helicobacter pylori* (*H. pylori*) antimicrobial resistance in Europe. *Gut* 39:A51.

Konturek SJ et al (1990) Role of prostaglandins in epidermal growth factor. *Dig Dis Sci* 33:1121.

Koo J et al (2001) Antacid increases survival of *Vibrio vulnificus* and *Vibrio vulnificus phage* in a gastrointestinal model. *Appl Environml Microbiol* 67: 2895–2902.

McCarthy DM (1991) Sucralfate. *N Engl J Med* 325(14):1017–1025.

Miller GD et al (2001) The importance of meeting calcium needs with foods. *Am J Clin Nutr* 20(2);168S–185S.

Mortensen L et al (1996) Bioavailability of calcium supplements and the effect of Vitamin D: Comparisons between milk, calcium carbonate, and calcium carbonate plus vitamin D. *Am J Clin Nutr* 63:354-357.

Nagashima R (1981) Development and characteristics of sucralfate. *J Clin Gastroentrol* 3:103–110.

Nicklas W (1992) Aluminum salts. *Res Immunol* 143:489.

NIH Consensus Development Panel on *H. pylori* in Peptic Ulcer Disease (1994) *Helicobacter pylori* in peptic ulcer disease. *JAMA* 272:65–69.

Peterson WI et al (1977) Healing of duodenal ulcer with antacid regimen. *N Engl J Med* 297:341.

Redd B et al (1996) Metronidazole resistance is high in Korea and Colombia and appears to be rapidly increasing in the U.S. *Gastroenterology* 10:A236.

Rubin JS and J Brasco (2003) *Restoring Your Digestive Health.* New York, NY: Kensington Publishing Corp; 47–48, 57–59.

Sachs G et al (1990) Gastric H + ,K + -ATPase as a therapeutic target in peptic ulcer disease. *Dig Dis Sci* 35:1537.

Sherrard DJ (1991) Aluminum—much ado about something. *N Engl J Med* 324:558.

Tani N (2003) Problems due to prolonged PPI use—other adverse effects, and safety. *Clin Gastreoenterol* 17:2.

Tarnawski A et al (1990) Antacids: New Perspectives in cytoprotection. *Scand J Gastroenterol Suppl* 174:9.

Thompson WG (1996) *The Ulcer Story.* New York, NY: Plenum Publishing Corp; 259–307.

Wagstaff AJ et al (1988) Colloidal bismuth subcitrate. A review of its pharmacodynamic and pharmacokinetic properties, and its therapeutic use in peptic ulcer disease. *Drugs* 36(2):132–157.

Walt RP (1992) Misoprostol for the treatment of peptic ulcer and anti-inflammatory-drug induced gastroduodenal ulceration. *N Eng J Med* 327:1575.

Chapter 7

Alberts DS et al (1996) Randomized, double-blind, placebo-controlled study of effect of wheat bran fiber and calcium on fecal bile acids in patients with resected adenomatous colon polyps. *J Natl Cancer Inst*, 88(2):81–92.

Al-Habbal MJ et al (1984) A double-blind controlled clinical trial of mastic and placebo in the treatment of duodenal ulcer. *Clin Exp Pharmacol Physiol* 11(5):541.

Al-Said MS et al (1986) Evaluation of mastic, a crude drug obtained from *Pistacia lentiscus* for gastric and duodenal anti-ulcer activity. *J Ethnopharmacol* 15(3):271–278.

Aydin A et al (2000) Garlic oil and *Helicobacter pylori* infection [letter]. *Am J Gastroenterol* 95:563–564.

Bergner P (2000) Garlic and *Helicobacter pylori* revisited. *Medical Herbalism* 11;2:10.

Bhatia SJ et al (1989) *Lactobacillus acidophilus* inhibits growth of *Campylobacter pylori in vitro*. *J Clin Microbiol* 27:2328–2330.

Canducci F et al (2000) A lyophilized and inactivated culture of *Lactobacillus acidophilus* increases *Helicobacter pylori* eradication rate. *Aliment Pharmacol Ther* 14:1625–1629.

Cheney G (1949) Rapid healing of peptic ulcers in patients receiving fresh cabbage juice. *Cal Med* 70:10.

Cheney G (1952) Vitamin U therapy for peptic ulcer. *Cal Med* 77;4:248–252.

Cheng Y et al (2000) Physical activity and peptic ulcers. *Western J Med* 173:101–107.

Editors (2002) News Summary. *Pharmaceutic J* 268;7192:453–457.

Ernst E (1999). Is garlic an effective treatment for *Helicobacter pylori* infection? *Arch Intern Med.* 159:2484–2485.

Fahey JW (2002) Sulforaphane inhibits extracellular, intracellular, and antibiotic-resistant strains of *Helicobacter pylori* and prevents benzo[a]pyrene-induced stomach tumors. *Proc Natl Acad Sci* 9(11):7610–5.

Fahey JW et al (1997) Broccoli sprouts: An exceptionally rich source of inducers of enzymes that protect against chemical carcinogens. *Proc Natl Acad Sci* 94:10367–10372.

Gaby AR (2001) *Helicobacter pylori* eradication: Are there alternatives to antibiotics? *Altern Med Rev* 6(4):355–366.

Graham DY (1999) Garlic or jalapeño peppers for treatment of *Helicobacter pylori* infection. *Amer J Gastroenterol* 94:1200–1202.

Huwez FU et al (1998) Mastic gum kills *Helicobacter pylori*. *N Engl J Med* 339:194–196.

Jarosz M et al (1998) Effects of high dose vitamin C treatment on *Helicobacter pylori* infection and total vitamin C concentration in gastric juice. *Eur J Cancer Prev* 7:449–454.

Kabir AM et al (1997) Prevention of *Helicobacter pylori* infection by lactobacilli in a gnotobiotic murine model. *Gut* 41:49–55.

Lee SH et al (2001) Vitamin C-induced decomposition of lipid hydroperoxides to endogenous genotoxins. *Science* 292(5524):2083–2086.

McArthur K et al (1982) Relative stimulatory effects of commonly ingested beverages on gastric acid secretion in humans. *Gastroenterol* 83:199.

Mrda Z (1998) Therapy of *Helicobacter pylori* infection using *Lactobacillus acidophilus*. *Med Pregl* 51(7–8):343–345.

Rees WD et al (1979) Effect of deglycyrrhizinated liquorice on gastric mucosal damage by aspirin. *Scand J Gastroenterol* 14(5):605–607.

Rubin JS and J Brasco (2003) *Restoring Your Digestive Health*. New York, NY: Kensington Publishing Corp; 121–123,190.

Simon JA et al (2003) Relation of serum ascorbic acid to *Helicobacter pylori* serology in US adults: The third national health and nutrition examination survey. *J Amer Coll Nutr* 22(4):283–289.

Stormer FC et al (1993) Glycyrrhizic acid in liquorice—evaluation of a health hazard. *Food Chem Toxic* 31:303–312.

Turpie AGG et al (1969) Clinical trials of deglycyrrhizinated liquorice in gastric ulcer. *Gut* 10:299–302.

Wang X et al (2000) Astaxanthin-rich algal meal and vitamin C inhibit *Helicobacter pylori* infection in balb/ca mice. *Antimicrob Agents Chemother* 44;9:2452-2457.

Weis R (2002) Study touts broccoli to fight ulcers, cancer. *Washington Post* May 28; A04.

Chapter 8

Amakawa T et al (1992) Clinical effect of Z-103 tablets against gastric ulcers: Phase III clinical study *Jpn Pharmacol Ther* 20(1):199–223.

Andrews M et al (1999) The role of zinc in wound healing. *Adv Wound Care* 12(3):137–138.

DiSilvestro R (2002) Review of studies relevant to the safety of use of Z-103. Data on file: FDA.

Fuji Y et al (2000) Protection by polaprezinc, an anti-ulcer drug, against indomethacin-induced apoptosis in rat gastric mucosal cells. *Jpn J Pharmacol* 84(1):63-70.

Furuta S et al (1999) Tissue distribution of polaprezinc in rats determined by the double tracer method. *J Pharm Biomed Anal* 19(3–4):453–461.

Hiraishi H et al (1999) Polaprezinc protects gastric mucosal cells from noxious agents through antioxidant properties *in vitro*. *Aliment Pharmacol Ther* 13(2):261–269.

Hojo M et al (2000) Do mucosal defensive agents improve the cure rate when used with dual or triple therapy regimens for eradicating *Helicobacter pylori* infection? *Aliment Pharmacol Ther* 14:193–201.

Hori Y et al The antioxidant properties of a novel anti-ulcer agent, Polaprezinc. Data on file: Zaria Pharm & 1st Dept Med, Kyoto Prefect U Med, Japan.

Kashimura H et al (1999) Polaprezinc, a mucosal protective agent, in combination with lansoprazole, amoxicillin and clarithromycin increases the cure rate of Helicobacter pylori infection. *Aliment Pharmacol Ther* 13:483–487.

Katayama S et al (2000) Effect of polaprezinc on healing of acetic acid-induced stomatitis in hamsters. *J Pharm Pharm Sci* 3(1):114–117.

Kato S et al (1997) Mucosal ulcerogenic action of monochloramine in rat stomachs: effects of polaprezinc and sucralfate. *Dig Dis Sci* 42(10):2156–2163.

Kato S et al (2001) Effect of polaprezinc on impaired healing of chronic gastric ulcers in adjuvant-induced arthritic rats—role of insulin-like growth factors (IGF)-1. *Med Sci Monit* 7(1):20–25.

Korolkiewicz RP et al (2000) Polaprezinc exerts a salutary effect on impaired healing of acute gastric lesions in diabetic rats. *Dig Dis Sci* 45(6):1200–1209.

Matsukura T (2000) Applicability of zinc complex of L-carnosine for medical use. *Biochemistry (Mosc)* 65(7):817–823.

Miyoshi A et al (1992) Clinical evaluation of Z-103 in the treatment of gastric ulcer: A multicenter double-blind dose finding study. *Jpn Pharm Ther* 20:181–197.

Naito Y (2001) Effects of polaprezinc on lipid peroxidation, neutrophil accumulation, and TNF-alpha expression in rats with aspirin-induced gastric mucosal injury. *Dig Dis Sci* 46(4):845–851.

Nishiwaki H et al (1997) Irritant action of monochloramine in rat stomachs: Effects of zinc L-carnosine (polaprezinc). *Gen Pharmacol* 29(5):713–718.

Pories WJ et al (1967) Acceleration of healing with zinc sulfate. *Ann Surg* 165:432–436.

Seiki M et al (992) The gastric mucosal adhesiveness of Z-103 in rats with chronic ulcer [article in Japanese] *Nippon Yakurigaku Zasshi* 99(4):255–263.

Seto K et al (1999) Effect of polaprezinc (N-(3-aminopropionyl)-L-histidinato zinc), a novel antiulcer agent containing zinc, on cellular proliferation: role of insulin-like growth factor I. *Biochem Pharmacol* 15;58(2): 245–250.

Shimada T et al (1999) Polaprezinc down-regulates proinflammatory cytokine-induced nuclear factor-kappaB activiation and interleukin-8 expression in gastric epithelial cells. *J Pharmacol Exp Ther* 291(1):345–352.

Sunairi M et al (1994) Effect of Z-103, a new antiulcer agent, on *Helicobacter pylori*. *Jpn Pharmacol Ther* 22:3771–3775.

Wollschlaeger B (2003) Zinc-carnosine for the management of gastric ulcers: Clinical application and literature review. *JANA* 6;2:32–39.

Yamaguchi I et al (1999) Toxic appearance and changes of zinc and copper contents in rats by long-term orally dosing of Z-103. Study undertaken by the Central Laboratory, Zeria Pharmaceutical Company.

Yoneta T et al (1994) Effects of polaprezinc (Z-103) on various acute experimental models of gastric and duodenal lesions in rats. *Ther Res* 15:4113–4121.

Yosikawa T et al (1991) The antioxidant properties of a novel zinc-carnosine chelate compound, N-(3-aminopropionyl)-L-histidinato zinc. *Biochim Biophys Acta* 1115:15–22.

Index

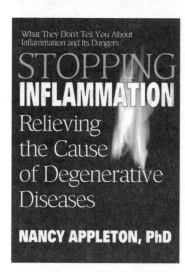

STOPPING INFLAMMATION

Relieving the Cause of Degenerative Diseases

Nancy Appleton, PhD

Most of us think of inflammation as a symptom associated with an infection or injury. Dr. Nancy Appleton, however, has discovered that it might be more than just a simple reaction to a health disorder. When the body's tissues are disturbed in some manner, a series of complex reactions takes place, resulting in inflammation. In most cases, when the disorder stops, the tissue returns to its normal healthy state. Sometimes, though, the tissue remains chronically inflamed. Dr. Appleton's early research demonstrated that this condition might be more harmful than ever suspected. Soon, she began to ask questions: What if inflammation was at the heart of various degenerative diseases? What health benefits could be gained if we could stop inflammation? *Stopping Inflammation* is the result of Dr. Appleton's quest to answer these important questions.

Drawing on the latest medical research, the book begins with a full explanation of inflammation and its causes. It then looks at its role in the various health disorders that afflict modern society, from obesity to heart disease to cancer. Finally, the book provides a number of nondrug treatments aimed not at controlling the problem, but at removing its cause.

Twenty years ago, Dr. Nancy Appleton's groundbreaking bestseller *Lick the Sugar Habit* exposed the dangers of ingesting excessive amounts of sugar. In *Stopping Inflammation,* Dr. Appleton examines the larger picture of twenty-first-century disease, and offers safe and credible solutions.

Nancy Appleton, PhD, earned her BS in clinical nutrition from UCLA and her PhD in health services from Walden University. She maintains a private practice in Santa Monica, California. An avid researcher, Dr. Appleton lectures throughout the world, and has appeared on numerous television and radio talk shows. She is the best-selling author of *Lick the Sugar Habit* and *Healthy Bones*.

$14.95 • 228 pages • 6 x 9-inch paperback • Health • ISBN 0-7570-0148-3

THE MAGNESIUM SOLUTION FOR HIGH BLOOD PRESSURE
How to Use Magnesium to Help Prevent and Relieve Hypertension Naturally
Jay S. Cohen, MD

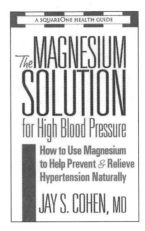

Approximately 50 percent of all Americans have hypertension, a devastating disease that can lead to hardening of the arteries, heart attack, and stroke. While many medications are available to combat this condition, these drugs come with potentially dangerous side effects. When Dr. Jay S. Cohen learned of his own hypertension, he was well aware of the risks associated with standard treatments. Based upon his research, he selected a safer option—magnesium.

In *The Magnesium Solution for High Blood Pressure,* Dr. Cohen describes the most effective types of magnesium for treating hypertension, explores appropriate magnesium dosage, and details the use of magnesium in conjunction with hypertension meds. Here is a proven remedy for anyone looking for a safe, effective approach to the treatment of high blood pressure.

$5.95 • 64 pages • 4 x 7.5-inch mass paperback • Health/High Blood Pressure • ISBN 0-7570-0255-2

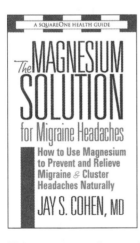

THE MAGNESIUM SOLUTION FOR MIGRAINE HEADACHES
How to Use Magnesium to Prevent and Relieve Migraine and Cluster Headaches Naturally
Jay S. Cohen, MD

More than 30 million people across North America suffer from migraine headaches. Over the years, a number of drugs have been developed to treat migraines, but these treatments don't work for everyone, and come with a high risk of side effects. Fortunately, Dr. Jay S. Cohen has discovered an alternative—magnesium.

This easy-to-understand guide explains what a migraine is, and shows how this supplement can play a key role in preventing and treating migraine headaches. It also describes what type of magnesium works best, and how much magnesium should be taken to prevent or stop migraines. For those who are looking for a safe and effective approach to the prevention and treatment of migraine and cluster headaches, Dr. Cohen prescribes a proven natural remedy in *The Magnesium Solution for Migraine Headaches.*

$5.95 • 64 pages • 4 x 7.5-inch mass paperback • Health/Migraines • ISBN 0-7570-0256-0

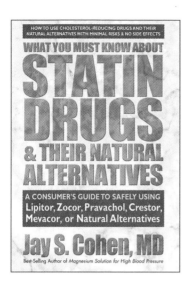

WHAT YOU MUST KNOW ABOUT STATIN DRUGS & THEIR NATURAL ALTERNATIVES

A Consumer's Guide to Safely Using Lipitor, Zocor, Pravachol, Crestor, Mevacor, or Natural Alternatives

Jay S. Cohen, MD

It is estimated that over 100 million Americans suffer from elevated cholesterol and C-reactive proteins—markers that are linked to heart attack, stroke, and other cardiovascular disorders. To combat these problems, modern science has created a group of drugs known either as statins or as specific commercial drugs such as Lipitor, Zocor, and Pravachol. While over 20 million people take these medications, the fact is that up to 42 percent experience side effects, and a whopping 60 to 70 percent eventually stop treatment. Here, for the first time, is a guide that explains the problems caused by statins, and offers easy-to-follow strategies that will allow you to benefit from these drugs while avoiding their side effects. In addition, the author provides natural alternatives that have also proven effective.

What You Must Know About Statin Drugs & Their Natural Alternatives begins by explaining elevated cholesterol and C-reactive proteins. It then examines how statins work to alleviate these problems, and discusses possible side effects. Highlighted is information on safe usage, as well as a discussion of effective alternative treatments. If you have elevated cholesterol and C-reactive proteins, or if you are currently using a statin, *What You Must Know About Statin Drugs & Their Natural Alternatives* can make a profound difference in the quality of your life.

Jay S. Cohen, MD, is an associate professor of family and preventive medicine and of psychiatry at the University of California, San Diego, where he teaches medical students and staff. For over thirteen years, Dr. Cohen specialized in psychopharmacology. Since 1990, he has conducted research on drugs and their side effects. He is the author of numerous research papers, published articles, and books, including *Over Dose: The Case Against the Drug Companies.* Dr. Cohen currently lives in Del Mar, California.

$15.95 • 204 pages • 6 x 9-inch paperback • Health • ISBN 0-7570-0257-9

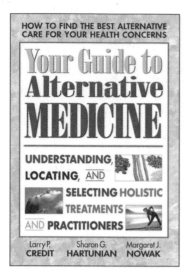

HOW TO FIND THE BEST ALTERNATIVE CARE FOR YOUR HEALTH CONCERNS

Your Guide to Alternative MEDICINE

UNDERSTANDING, LOCATING, AND SELECTING HOLISTIC TREATMENTS AND PRACTITIONERS

Larry P. **CREDIT**   Sharon G. **HARTUNIAN**   Margaret J. **NOWAK**

Your Guide to Alternative Medicine

Understanding, Locating, and Selecting Holistic Treatments and Practitioners

Larry P. Credit, Sharon G. Hartunian, and Margaret J. Nowak

The growing world of complementary medicine offers safe and effective solutions to many health disorders, from backache to headache. You may already be interested in alternative care approaches, but if you're like most people, you have a hundred and one questions you'd like answered before you choose a treatment. "Will I feel the acupuncture needles?" "What is a homeopathic remedy?" "Does chiropractic hurt?" *Your Guide to Alternative Medicine* provides the fundamental facts necessary to choose an effective complementary care therapy and begin treatment.

This comprehensive reference clearly explains numerous approaches in an easy-to-read format. For every complementary care option discussed, there is a description and brief history; a list of conditions that respond; information on the cost and duration of treatment; credentials and educational background for practitioners; and more. To find those therapies most appropriate for a specific condition, there is even a unique troubleshooting chart.

Your Guide to Alternative Medicine introduces you to options that you may never have considered—techniques that enhance the body's natural healing potential and have few, if any, side effects. Here is a reference that can help you make informed decisions about all your important healthcare needs.

$11.95 • 208 pages • 6 x 9-inch quality paperback • Health/Alternative Therapies/Reference ISBN 0-7570-0125-4